CONTENTS

INTRODUCTION

A Brief of The Pit Boss Wood Pellet Grill

Pit Boss Grills is a subsidiary of Dansons, Inc. which was founded in 1999 by Dan Thiessen and his two sons, Jeff and Jordan. Pit Boss Grills is known for their durability and craftsmanship, as well as for their family style and approach to business. From portable grills like the Pit Boss Tailgater, to massive grills like the Pit Boss Austin XL – Pit Boss Grills takes pride in creating whatever the customers (and employees) dream up. Last year, Dansons was awarded EY Entrepreneur of the Year (2017). Today, Pit Boss Grills are the best value per square inch in the market, and pellet grills are the fastest growing segment within that market. Being Bigger. Hotter. Heavier. than the competition at a better value, and constantly striving to improve, are two of the founding principles Pit Boss was built upon. Creating a community around outdoor cooking, backyard barbeques, and neighborhood block parties is an idea Pit Boss is proud to be a part of, and proud to be included in.

What is The Pit Boss Wood Pellet Grill?

Pit Boos Wood-pellet grills give you the flavor of food cooked over hardwood while allowing for good temperature control. Pellet grills are extremely versatile,with temps up to 500 degrees, and a "low-and-slow" smoker. And both brands come equipped with digital controllers for a more accurate temperature setting.Pellet grills also let you subtly flavor your food with different types of wood pellets. Both and Pit Boss sell their own brand of pellets with their own mix of wood flavors. Pit Boss pellets have more of a reputation for turning to unusable sawdust, but overall people don't have a problem with them, and they are cheaper than pellets. When deciding which pellet grill to buy, the first thing to consider is size. Both and Pit Boss sell many sizes, but if you're looking for very small or very large grills, has a wider range of cooking space available. You'll also want to consider the mobility of your grill. Will you want to pack it for a tailgating party or bring it fishing? Both brands make portable grills, but Traeger's lineup includes smaller, easier-to-move options.

How to Use Your Pit Boss Wood Pellet Grill?

Any Pit Boss grill gives you a function called Priming - this is important because it gives you manual control of the speed of the Auger.So when the pellets have run out or you're starting your first grill, there are no pellets lined up in the auger to be fed to the ignitor which starts your fire. When the grill starts, it runs the auger and igniter for 4 minutes straight no matter what. If the pellets don't reach the ignitor in time, no fire will start. Make SURE you PRIME by holding down the prime button until you hear pellets drop into the fire pot, or see smoke. You will hear the trickling, like dropping a penny into a soda can.

As for the P Setting...

P0 = FASTEST

P4 = Default

P7 = SLOWEST

If it were the middle of the unforgiving Alaskan winter, (which a Pit Boss will still run in) you would want to try a P Setting of 0 to counter the naturally frigid winter air and outside temperatures. On the other hand, if you were cooking in the Sahara dessert, your grill might already by 200 degrees inside from the stifling dessert sun.

FAQs on Your Pit Boss Wood Pellet Grill

Should you leave your Pit Boss outside?

Note that if you leave your grill outside, you should cover it properly to avoid water damage. Maintaining and caring for your grill will keep it in tip-top shape for longer. When it comes to design and construction, not many models can match the Pit Boss. Most of the grills come with amazing features like cast-iron grates, with a non-toxic coating that prevents your food from sticking to the grates. In addition, the fireboxes come with similar materials. Although the other wood pellet grills come with similar elements, most of them look flimsy, and most of them will not meet your smoking and grilling demands

What is the smoke setting on Pit Boss smokers?

Smokers come with a factory preset temperature of 160-190 degrees on smoke mode. This temperature is ideal for smoking most meats. The smoke setting or P setting is 225 degrees Fahrenheit. Note that P settings are for smoking, not cooking.

VEGETABLE & VEGETARIAN RECIPES

1.   Smoked 3-bean Salad

Servings: 6
Cooking Time: 20 Minutes
Ingredients:
- 1 can Great Northern Beans, rinsed and drained
- 1 can Red Kidney Beans, rinsed and drained
- 1pound fresh green beans, trimmed
- 2 tablespoons olive oil
- Salt and pepper to taste
- 1 shallot, sliced thinly
- 2 tablespoons red wine vinegar
- 1 teaspoon Dijon mustard

Directions:
1.   Fire the Grill to 500F. Use desired wood pellets when cooking. Close the lid and preheat for 15 minutes.
2.   Place the beans in a sheet tray and drizzle with olive oil. Season with salt and pepper to taste.
3.   Place in the grill and cook for 20 minutes. Make sure to shake the tray for even cooking.
4.   Once cooked, remove the beans and place in a bowl. Allow to cool first.
5.   Add the shallots and the rest of the ingredients. Season with more salt and pepper if desired. Toss to coat the beans with the seasoning.

Nutrition Info: Calories per serving: 179; Protein: 8.2 g; Carbs: 23.5g; Fat: 6.5g Sugar: 2.2g

2.   Roasted Green Beans With Bacon

Servings: 6

Cooking Time: 20 Minutes

Ingredients:

- 1-pound green beans
- 4 strips bacon, cut into small pieces
- 4 tablespoons extra virgin olive oil
- 2 cloves garlic, minced
- 1 teaspoon salt

Directions:

1. Fire the Grill to 400F. Use desired wood pellets when cooking. Close the lid and preheat for 15 minutes.
2. Toss all ingredients on a sheet tray and spread out evenly.
3. Place the tray on the grill grate and roast for 20 minutes.

Nutrition Info: Calories per serving: 65 ; Protein: 1.3g; Carbs: 3.8g; Fat: 5.3g Sugar: 0.6g

3. Smoked Eggs

Servings: 12

Cooking Time: 30 Minutes

Ingredients:

- 12 hardboiled eggs, peeled and rinsed

Directions:

1. Supply your smoker with wood pellets and follow the manufacturer's specific start-up procedure. Preheat the grill, with the lid closed, to 120°F.

2. Place the eggs directly on the grill grate and smoke for 30 minutes. They will begin to take on a slight brown sheen.

3. Remove the eggs and refrigerate for at least 30 minutes before serving. Refrigerate any leftovers in an airtight container for 1 or 2 weeks.

4.   Smoked Pumpkin Soup

Servings: 6

Cooking Time: 1 Hour And 33 Minutes

Ingredients:

- 5 pounds pumpkin, seeded and sliced
- 3 tablespoons butter
- 1 onion, diced
- 2 cloves garlic, minced
- 1 tablespoon brown sugar
- 1 teaspoon paprika
- ¼ teaspoon ground cinnamon
- ¼ teaspoon ground nutmeg
- ½ cup apple cider
- 5 cups broth
- ½ cup cream

Directions:

1.   Fire the Grill to 180F. Use desired wood pellets when cooking. Close the lid and preheat for 15 minutes.

2.   Place the pumpkin on the grill grate and smoke for an hour or until tender. Allow to cool.

3.   Melt the butter in a large saucepan over medium heat and sauté the onion and garlic for 3 minutes. Stir in the rest of the ingredients including the smoked pumpkin. Cook for another 30 minutes.

4.   Transfer to a blender and pulse until smooth.

Nutrition Info: Calories per serving: 246; Protein: 8.8g; Carbs: 32.2g; Fat: 11.4g Sugar: 15.5g

5. Grilled Scallions

Servings: 6

Cooking Time: 20 Minutes

Ingredients:

- 10 whole scallions, chopped
- ¼ cup olive oil
- Salt and pepper to taste
- 2 tablespoons rice vinegar
- 1 whole jalapeno, sliced into rings

Directions:

1.   Fire the Grill to 500F. Use desired wood pellets when cooking. Close the lid and preheat for 15 minutes.

2.   Place on a bowl all ingredients and toss to coat. Transfer to a parchment-lined baking tray.

3.   Place on the grill grate and cook for 20 minutes or until the scallions char.

Nutrition Info: Calories per serving: 135; Protein: 2.2 g; Carbs: 9.7 g; Fat: 10.1g Sugar: 4.6g

6. Grilled Zucchini Squash Spears

Servings: 4

Cooking Time: 10 Minutes

Ingredients:

- 4 zucchini, medium
- 2 tbsp olive oil
- 1 tbsp sherry vinegar
- 2 thyme, leaves pulled
- Salt to taste
- Pepper to taste

Directions:

1. Clean zucchini, cut ends off, half each lengthwise, and cut each half into thirds.
2. Combine all the other ingredients in a zip lock bag, medium, then add spears.
3. Toss well and mix to coat the zucchini.
4. Preheat to 350F with the lid closed for about 15 minutes.
5. Remove spears from the zip lock bag and place them directly on your grill grate with the cut side down.
6. Cook for about 3-4 minutes until zucchini is tender and grill marks show.
7. Remove them from the grill and enjoy.

Nutrition Info: Calories 93, Total fat 7.4g, Saturated fat 1.1g, Total carbs 7.1g, Net carbs 4.9g, Protein 2.4g, Sugars 3.4g, Fiber 2.2g, Sodium 59mg, Potassium 515mg

7.   **Vegan Smoked Carrot Dogs**

Servings: 2

Cooking Time: 35 Minutes

Ingredients:

- 4 carrots, thick
- 2 tbsp avocado oil
- 1/2 tbsp garlic powder
- 1 tbsp liquid smoke
- Pepper to taste
- Kosher salt to taste

Directions:

1. Preheat your to 425F then line a parchment paper on a baking sheet.
2. Peel the carrots to resemble a hot dog. Round the edges when peeling.
3. Whisk together oil, garlic powder, liquid smoke, pepper and salt in a bowl, small.
4. Now place carrots on the baking sheet and pour the mixture over. Roll your carrots in the mixture to massage seasoning and oil into them. Use fingertips.
5. Roast the carrots in the until fork tender for about 35 minutes. Brush the carrots using the marinade mixture every 5 minutes.
6. Remove and place into hot dog buns then top with hot dog toppings of your choice.
7. Serve and enjoy!

Nutrition Info: Calories 76, Total fat 1.8g, Saturated 0.4g, Total 14.4g, Net carbs 10.6g, Protein 1.5g, Sugar 6.6g, Fiber 3.8g, Sodium 163mg, Potassium 458mg

8.   Sweet Potato Fries

Servings: 4

Cooking Time: 40 Minutes

Ingredients:

- 3 sweet potatoes, sliced into strips
- 4 tablespoons olive oil
- 2 tablespoons fresh rosemary, chopped
- Salt and pepper to taste

Directions:

1. Set the wood pellet grill to 450 degrees F.
2. Preheat it for 10 minutes.
3. Spread the sweet potato strips in the baking pan.
4. Toss in olive oil and sprinkle with rosemary, salt and pepper.
5. Cook for 15 minutes.
6. Flip and cook for another 15 minutes.
7. Flip and cook for 10 more minutes.
8. Tips: Soak sweet potatoes in water before cooking to prevent browning.

9.   Grilled Artichokes

Servings: 6

Cooking Time: 15 Minutes

Ingredients:

- 3 large artichokes, blanched and halved
- 3 + 3 tablespoons olive oil
- Salt and pepper to taste
- 1 cup mayonnaise
- 1 cup yogurt
- 2 tablespoons parsley, chopped
- 2 tablespoons capers
- Lemon juice to taste

Directions:

1.   Fire the Grill to 500F. Use desired wood pellets when cooking. Close the lid and preheat for 15 minutes.
2.   Brush the artichokes with 3 tablespoons of olive oil. Season with salt and pepper to taste.
3.   Place on the grill grate and cook for 15 minutes.
4.   Allow to cool before slicing.
5.   Once cooled, slice the artichokes and place in a bowl.
6.   In another bowl, mix together the mayonnaise, yogurt, parsley, capers, and lemon juice. Season with salt and pepper to taste. Mix until well-combined.
7.   Pour sauce over the artichokes.
8.   Toss to coat.

Nutrition Info: Calories per serving: 257; Protein: 6.7g; Carbs: 13.2 g; Fat: 20.9g Sugar: 3.7g

10.   Scampi Spaghetti Squash

Servings: 4
Cooking Time: 40 Minutes

Ingredients:

- 1 spaghetti squash
- 2 tablespoons extra-virgin olive oil
- 1 teaspoon salt
- 1 teaspoon freshly ground black pepper
- 2 teaspoons garlic powder
- 4 tablespoons (½ stick) unsalted butter
- ½ cup white wine
- 1 tablespoon minced garlic
- 2 teaspoons chopped fresh parsley
- 1 teaspoon red pepper flakes
- ½ teaspoon salt
- ½ teaspoon freshly ground black pepper

Directions:

1.   For the squash:
2.   Supply your smoker with wood pellets and follow the manufacturer's specific start-up procedure. Preheat, with the lid closed, to 375°F.
3.   Cut off both ends of the squash, then cut it in half lengthwise. Scoop out and discard the seeds.
4.   Rub the squash flesh well with the olive oil and sprinkle on the salt, pepper, and garlic powder.
5.   Place the squash cut-side up on the grill grate, close the lid, and smoke for 40 minutes, or until tender
6.   For the sauce:
7.   On the stove top, in a medium saucepan over medium heat, combine the butter, white wine, minced garlic, parsley, red pepper flakes, salt, and pepper, and cook for about 5 minutes, or until heated through. Reduce the heat to low and keep the sauce warm.
8.   Remove the squash from the grill and let cool slightly before shredding the flesh with a fork; discard the skin.
9.   Stir the shredded squash into the garlic-wine butter sauce and serve immediately.

11.   Blt Pasta Salad

Servings: 6
Cooking Time: 35 To 45 Minutes
Ingredients:
- 1 pound thick-cut bacon
- 16 ounces bowtie pasta, cooked according to package directions and drained
- 2 tomatoes, chopped
- ½ cup chopped scallions
- ½ cup Italian dressing
- ½ cup ranch dressing
- 1 tablespoon chopped fresh basil
- 1 teaspoon salt
- 1 teaspoon freshly ground black pepper
- 1 teaspoon garlic powder
- 1 head lettuce, cored and torn

Directions:
1. Supply your smoker with wood pellets and follow the manufacturer's specific start-up procedure. Preheat, with the lid closed, to 225°F.
2. Arrange the bacon slices on the grill grate, close the lid, and cook for 30 to 45 minutes, flipping after 20 minutes, until crisp.
3. Remove the bacon from the grill and chop.
4. In a large bowl, combine the chopped bacon with the cooked pasta, tomatoes, scallions, Italian dressing, ranch dressing, basil, salt, pepper, and garlic powder. Refrigerate until ready to serve.
5. Toss in the lettuce just before serving to keep it from wilting.

12.   Ramen Soup

Servings: 2

Cooking Time: 35 Minutes

Ingredients:

- 4cups Chicken Stock
- 1tbsp. Extra Virgin Olive Oil
- 2Baby Bok Choy Head, leaves torn
- 1Shallot, chopped into 1-inch piece
- 3oz. Ramen, dried
- 4Garlic cloves
- 1tsp. Sesame Oil, toasted
- 2tsp. Ginger, fresh
- One bunch of Green Onion, sliced thinly
- 1cup Chicken, cooked and cut into 1-inch cubes

Directions:

1. First, keep the olive oil, shallot, garlic, and ginger in the blender pitcher.
2. After that, press the 'saute' button.
3. Next, stir in the chicken, green onions, chicken stock, and sesame oil into it.
4. Now, select the 'hearty soup' button.
5. Then, three minutes before the program ends, spoon in the ramen noodles and baby bok choy.
6. Check the chicken's internal temperature and ensure it is 165 ° F and if it is, then transfer the soup to the serving bowls.
7. Serve immediately and enjoy it.

Nutrition Info: Calories: 190 Fat: 8g Total Carbs: 25g Fiber: 1 g Sugar: 0.5 g Protein: 3 g Cholesterol: 2.5 mg

13. **Stuffed Grilled Zucchini**

Servings: 4

Cooking Time: 10 Minutes

Ingredients:

- 4 zucchini, medium
- 5 tbsp olive oil, divided
- 2 tbsp red onion, finely chopped
- 1/4 tbsp garlic, minced
- 1/2 cup bread crumbs, dry
- 1/2 cup shredded mozzarella cheese, part-skim
- 1/2 tbsp salt
- 1 tbsp fresh mint, minced
- 3 tbsp parmesan cheese, grated

Directions:

1. Halve zucchini lengthwise and scoop pulp ou. Leave 1/4 -inch shell. Now brush using 2 tbsp oil, set aside, and chop the pulp.
2. Saute onion and pulp in a skillet, large, then add garlic and cook for about 1 minute.
3. Add bread crumbs and cook while stirring for about 2 minutes until golden brown.
4. Remove everything from heat then stir in mozzarella cheese, salt, and mint. Scoop into the zucchini shells and splash with parmesan cheese.
5. Preheat your to 375F.
6. Place stuffed zucchini on the grill and grill while covered for about 8-10 minutes until tender.
7. Serve warm and enjoy.

Nutrition Info: Calories 186, Total fat 10g, Saturated fat 3g, Total carbs 17g, Net carbs 14g, Protein 9g, Sugars 4g, Fiber 3g, Sodium 553mg, Potassium 237mg

14.   Zucchini Soup

Servings: 4
Cooking Time: 35 Minutes
Ingredients:
- 2tbsp. Olive Oil
- 1lb. Zucchini, chopped coarsely
- 1Onion quartered
- 8 oz. Watercress, chopped
- Salt and Black Pepper, as needed
- Pinch of Saffron
- 3cups Chicken Broth
- 1tbsp. Heavy Cream

Directions:
1. First, place olive oil and onion in the blender pitcher and press the 'saute' button.
2. Once sautéed, add all the remaining ingredients to it.
3. Now, press the 'smooth soup' button.
4. Finally, transfer the soup to the serving bowls and serve immediately.

Nutrition Info: Calories: 249 Fat: 20 g Total Carbs: 15 g Fiber: 4.1 g Sugar: 10 g Protein: 4.9 g Cholesterol: 15 mg

15.   Grilled Zucchini Squash

Servings: 6

Cooking Time: 10 Minutes

Ingredients:

- 3 medium zucchinis, sliced into ¼ inch thick lengthwise
- 2 tablespoons olive oil
- 1 tablespoon sherry vinegar
- 2 thyme leaves, pulled
- Salt and pepper to taste

Directions:

1.   Fire the Grill to 350F. Use desired wood pellets when cooking. Close the lid and preheat for 15 minutes.

2.   Place zucchini in a bowl and all ingredients. Gently massage the zucchini slices to coat with the seasoning.

3.   Place the zucchini on the grill grate and cook for 5 minutes on each side.

Nutrition Info: Calories per serving: 44; Protein: 0.3 g; Carbs: 0.9 g; Fat: 4g Sugar: 0.1g

16.   Georgia Sweet Onion Bake

Servings: 6

Cooking Time: 1 Hour

Ingredients:

- Nonstick cooking spray or butter, for greasing
- 4 large Vidalia or other sweet onions
- 8 tablespoons (1 stick) unsalted butter, melted
- 4 chicken bouillon cubes
- 1 cup grated Parmesan cheese

Directions:

1.   Supply your smoker with wood pellets and follow the manufacturer's specific start-up procedure. Preheat, with the lid closed, to 350°F.

2.   Coat a high-sided baking pan with cooking spray or butter.

3.   Peel the onions and cut into quarters, separating into individual petals.

4.   Spread the onions out in the prepared pan and pour the melted butter over them.

5.   Crush the bouillon cubes and sprinkle over the buttery onion pieces, then top with the cheese.

6.   Transfer the pan to the grill, close the lid, and smoke for 30 minutes.

7.   Remove the pan from the grill, cover tightly with aluminum foil, and poke several holes all over to vent.

8.   Place the pan back on the grill, close the lid, and smoke for an additional 30 to 45 minutes.

9.   Uncover the onions, stir, and serve hot.

17.   Cauliflower With Parmesan And Butter

Servings: 4

Cooking Time: 45 Minutes

Ingredients:

- 1 medium head of cauliflower
- 1 teaspoon minced garlic
- 1 teaspoon salt
- ½ teaspoon ground black pepper
- 1/4 cup olive oil
- 1/2 cup melted butter, unsalted
- 1/2 tablespoon chopped parsley
- 1/4 cup shredded parmesan cheese

Directions:

1.   Switch on the grill, fill the grill hopper with flavored wood pellets, power the grill on by using the control panel, select 'smoke' on the temperature dial, or set the temperature to 450 degrees F and let it preheat for a minimum of 15 minutes.

2.   Meanwhile, brush the cauliflower head with oil, season with salt and black pepper and then place in a skillet pan.

3.   When the grill has preheated, open the lid, place prepared skillet pan on the grill grate, shut the grill and smoke for 45 minutes until golden brown and the center has turned tender.

4.   Meanwhile, take a small bowl, place melted butter in it, and then stir in garlic, parsley, and cheese until combined.

5.   Baste cheese mixture frequently in the last 20 minutes of cooking and, when done, remove the pan from heat and garnish cauliflower with parsley.

6.   Cut it into slices and then serve.

Nutrition Info: Calories: 128 Cal ;Fat: 7.6 g ;Carbs: 10.8 g ;Protein: 7.4 g ;Fiber: 5 g

18.   Wood Pellet Grilled Stuffed Zucchini

Servings: 8

Cooking Time: 11 Minutes

Ingredients:

- 4 zucchini
- 5 tbsp olive oil
- 2 tbsp red onion, chopped
- 1/4 tbsp garlic, minced
- 1/2 cup bread crumbs
- 1/2 cup mozzarella cheese, shredded
- 1 tbsp fresh mint
- 1/2 tbsp salt
- 3 tbsp parmesan cheese

Directions:

1. Cut the zucchini lengthwise and scoop out the pulp then brush the shells with oil.
2. In a non-stick skillet sauté pulp, onion, and remaining oil. Add garlic and cook for a minute.
3. Add bread crumbs and cook until golden brown. Remove from heat and stir in mozzarella cheese, fresh mint, and salt.
4. Spoon the mixture into the shells and sprinkle parmesan cheese.
5. Place in a grill and grill for 10 minutes or until the zucchini are tender.

Nutrition Info: Calories 186, Total fat 10g, Saturated fat 5g, Total Carbs 17g, Net Carbs 14g, Protein 9g, Sugar 4g, Fiber 3g, Sodium: 553mg

19.   Bunny Dogs With Sweet And Spicy Jalapeño Relish

Servings: 8

Cooking Time: 35 To 40 Minutes

Ingredients:

- 8 hot dog-size carrots, peeled
- ¼ cup honey
- ¼ cup yellow mustard
- Nonstick cooking spray or butter, for greasing
- Salt
- Freshly ground black pepper
- 8 hot dog buns
- Sweet and Spicy Jalapeño Relish

Directions:

1. Prepare the carrots by removing the stems and slicing in half lengthwise.
2. In a small bowl, whisk together the honey and mustard.
3. Supply your smoker with wood pellets and follow the manufacturer's specific start-up procedure. Preheat, with the lid closed, to 375°F.
4. Line a baking sheet with aluminum foil and coat with cooking spray.
5. Brush the carrots on both sides with the honey mustard and season with salt and pepper; put on the baking sheet.
6. Place the baking sheet on the grill grate, close the lid, and smoke for 35 to 40 minutes, or until tender and starting to brown.
7. To serve, lightly toast the hot dog buns on the grill and top each with two slices of carrot and some relish.

20.   Whole Roasted Cauliflower With Garlic Parmesan Butter

Servings: 5
Cooking Time: 45 Minutes

Ingredients:

- 1/4 cup olive oil
- Salt and pepper to taste
- 1 cauliflower, fresh
- 1/2 cup butter, melted
- 1/4 cup parmesan cheese, grated
- 2 garlic cloves, minced
- 1/2 tbsp parsley, chopped

Directions:

1. Preheat the wood pellet grill with the lid closed for 15 minutes.
2. Meanwhile, brush the cauliflower with oil then season with salt and pepper.
3. Place the cauliflower in a cast iron and place it on a grill grate.
4. Cook for 45 minutes or until the cauliflower is golden brown and tender.
5. Meanwhile, mix butter, cheese, garlic, and parsley in a mixing bowl.
6. In the last 20 minutes of cooking, add the butter mixture.
7. Remove the cauliflower from the grill and top with more cheese and parsley if you desire. Enjoy.

Nutrition Info: Calories 156, Total fat 11.1g, Saturated fat 3.4g, Total Carbs 8.8g, Net Carbs 5.1g, Protein 8.2g, Sugar 0g, Fiber 3.7g, Sodium: 316mg, Potassium 468.2mg

21. Coconut Bacon

Servings: 2

Cooking Time: 30 Minutes

Ingredients:

- 3 1/2 cups flaked coconut
- 1 tbsp pure maple syrup
- 1 tbsp water
- 2 tbsp liquid smoke
- 1 tbsp soy sauce
- 1 tsp smoked paprika (optional)

Directions:

1. Preheat the smoker at 325°F.
2. Take a large mixing bowl and combine liquid smoke, maple syrup, soy sauce, and water.
3. Pour flaked coconut over the mixture. Add it to a cooking sheet.
4. Place in the middle rack of the smoker.
5. Smoke it for 30 minutes and every 7-8 minutes, keep flipping the sides.
6. Serve and enjoy.

Nutrition Info: Calories: 1244 Cal Fat: 100 g Carbohydrates: 70 g   Protein: 16 g Fiber: 2 g

22.   Wood Pellet Grilled Asparagus And Honey Glazed Carrots

Servings: 5

Cooking Time: 35 Minutes

Ingredients:

- 1 bunch asparagus, trimmed ends
- 1 lb carrots, peeled
- 2 tbsp olive oil
- Sea salt to taste
- 2 tbsp honey
- Lemon zest

Directions:

1.   Sprinkle the asparagus with oil and sea salt. Drizzle the carrots with honey and salt.
2.   Preheat the wood pellet to 165°F wit the lid closed for 15 minutes.
3.   Place the carrots in the wood pellet and cook for 15 minutes. Add asparagus and cook for 20 more minutes or until cooked through.
4.   Top the carrots and asparagus with lemon zest. Enjoy.

Nutrition Info: Calories 1680, Total fat 30g, Saturated fat 2g, Total Carbs 10g, Net Carbs 10g, Protein 4g, Sugar 0g, Fiber 0g, Sodium: 514mg, Potassium 0mg

23.   Roasted Hasselback Potatoes

Servings: 6
Cooking Time: 30 Minutes
Ingredients:
- 6 large russet potatoes
- 1-pound bacon
- ½ cup butter
- Salt to taste
- 1 cup cheddar cheese
- 3 whole scallions, chopped

Directions:
1.   Fire the Grill to 350F. Use desired wood pellets when cooking. Close the lid and preheat for 15 minutes.
2.   Place two wooden spoons on either side of the potato and slice the potato into thin strips without completely cutting through the potato.
3.   Chop the bacon into small pieces and place in between the cracks or slices of the potatoes.
4.   Place potatoes in a cast iron skillet. Top the potatoes with butter, salt, and cheddar cheese.
5.   Place the skillet on the grill grate and cook for 30 minutes. Make sure to baste the potatoes with melted cheese 10 minutes before the cooking time ends.
Nutrition Info: Calories per serving: 662; Protein: 16.1g; Carbs: 71.5g; Fat: 38g Sugar: 2.3g

Servings: 6
Cooking Time: 45 Minutes

Ingredients:
- 16 to 20 long toothpicks
- 1 pound Brussels sprouts, trimmed and wilted, leaves removed
- ½ pound bacon, cut in half
- 1 tablespoon packed brown sugar
- 1 tablespoon Cajun seasoning
- ¼ cup balsamic vinegar
- ¼ cup extra-virgin olive oil
- ¼ cup chopped fresh cilantro
- 2 teaspoons minced garlic

Directions:
1. Soak the toothpicks in water for 15 minutes.
2. Supply your smoker with wood pellets and follow the manufacturer's specific start-up procedure. Preheat, with the lid closed, to 300°F.
3. Wrap each Brussels sprout in a half slice of bacon and secure with a toothpick.
4. In a small bowl, combine the brown sugar and Cajun seasoning. Dip each wrapped Brussels sprout in this sweet rub and roll around to coat.
5. Place the sprouts on a Frogmat or parchment paper–lined baking sheet on the grill grate, close the lid, and smoke for 45 minutes to 1 hour, turning as needed, until cooked evenly and the bacon is crisp.
6. In a small bowl, whisk together the balsamic vinegar, olive oil, cilantro, and garlic.
7. Remove the toothpicks from the Brussels sprouts, transfer to a plate and serve drizzled with the cilantro-balsamic sauce.

25.   Smoked And Smashed New Potatoes

Servings: 4

Cooking Time: 8 Hours

Ingredients:

- 1-1/2 pounds small new red potatoes or fingerlings
- Extra virgin olive oil
- Sea salt and black pepper
- 2 tbsp softened butter

Directions:

1. Let the potatoes dry. Once dried, put in a pan and coat with salt, pepper, and extra virgin olive oil.
2. Place the potatoes on the topmost rack of the smoker.
3. Smoke for 60 minutes.
4. Once done, take them out and smash each one
5. Mix with butter and season

Nutrition Info: Calories: 258 Cal Fat: 2.0 g Carbohydrates: 15.5 g   Protein: 4.1 g Fiber: 1.5 g

26.   Vegetable Skewers

Servings: 4
Cooking Time: 20 Minutes

Ingredients:

- 2 cups whole white mushrooms
- 2 large yellow squash, peeled, chopped
- 1 cup chopped pineapple
- 1 cup chopped red pepper
- 1 cup halved strawberries
- 2 large zucchini, chopped
- For the Dressing:
- 2 lemons, juiced
- ½ teaspoon ground black pepper
- 1/2 teaspoon sea salt
- 1 teaspoon red chili powder
- 1 tablespoon maple syrup
- 1 tablespoon orange zest
- 2 tablespoons apple cider vinegar
- 1/4 cup olive oil

Directions:

1.   Switch on the grill, fill the grill hopper with flavored wood pellets, power the grill on by using the control panel, select 'smoke' on the temperature dial, or set the temperature to 450 degrees F and let it preheat for a minimum of 5 minutes.

2.   Meanwhile, prepared thread vegetables and fruits on skewers alternately and then brush skewers with oil.

3.   When the grill has preheated, open the lid, place vegetable skewers on the grill grate, shut the grill, and smoke for 20 minutes until tender and lightly charred.

4.   Meanwhile, prepare the dressing and for this, take a small bowl, place all of its ingredients in it and then whisk until combined.

5.   When done, transfer skewers to a dish, top with prepared dressing and then serve.

Nutrition Info: Calories: 130 Cal ;Fat: 2 g ;Carbs: 20 g ;Protein: 2 g ;Fiber: 0.3 g

FISH AND SEAFOOD RECIPES

27.   Jerk Shrimp

Servings: 12
Cooking Time: 6 Minutes
Ingredients:
- 2 pounds shrimp, peeled, deveined
- 3 tablespoons olive oil
- For the Spice Mix:
- 1 teaspoon garlic powder
- 1 teaspoon of sea salt
- 1/4 teaspoon ground cayenne
- 1 tablespoon brown sugar
- 1/8 teaspoon smoked paprika
- 1 tablespoon smoked paprika
- 1/4 teaspoon ground thyme
- 1 lime, zested

Directions:
1.   Switch on the grill, fill the grill hopper with flavored wood pellets, power the grill on by using the control panel, select 'smoke' on the temperature dial, or set the temperature to 450 degrees F and let it preheat for a minimum of 5 minutes.
2.   Meanwhile, prepare the spice mix and for this, take a small bowl, place all of its ingredients in it and stir until mixed.
3.   Take a large bowl, place shrimps in it, sprinkle with prepared spice mix, drizzle with oil and toss until well coated.
4.   When the grill has preheated, open the lid, place shrimps on the grill grate, shut the grill and smoke for 3 minutes per side until firm and thoroughly cooked.
5.   When done, transfer shrimps to a dish and then serve.
Nutrition Info: Calories: 131 Cal ;Fat: 4.3 g ;Carbs: 0 g ;Protein: 22 g ;Fiber: 0 g

28. Grilled Blackened Salmon

Servings: 4

Cooking Time: 30 Minutes

Ingredients:

- 4 salmon fillet
- Blackened dry rub
- Italian seasoning powder

Directions:

1. Season salmon fillets with dry rub and seasoning powder.
2. Grill in the wood pellet grill at 325 degrees F for 10 to 15 minutes per side.
3. Tips: You can also drizzle salmon with lemon juice

29.   Lively Flavored Shrimp

Servings: 6

Cooking Time: 30 Minutes

Ingredients:

- 8 oz. salted butter, melted
- ¼ C. Worcestershire sauce
- ¼ C. fresh parsley, chopped
- 1 lemon, quartered
- 2 lb. jumbo shrimp, peeled and deveined
- 3 tbsp. BBQ rub

Directions:

1. In a metal baking pan, add all ingredients except for shrimp and BBQ rub and mix well.
2. Season the shrimp with BBQ rub evenly.
3. Add the shrimp in the pan with butter mixture and coat well.
4. Set aside for about 20-30 minutes.
5. Set the temperature of Grill to 250 degrees F and preheat with closed lid for 15 minutes.
6. Place the pan onto the grill and cook for about 25-30 minutes.
7. Remove the pan from grill and serve hot.

Nutrition Info: Calories per serving: 462; Carbohydrates: 4.7g; Protein: 34.9g; Fat: 33.3g; Sugar: 2.1g; Sodium: 485mg; Fiber: 0.2g

30. Smoked Scallops

Servings: 6
Cooking Time: 15 Minutes

Ingredients:

- 2 pounds sea scallops
- 4 tbsp salted butter
- 2 tbsp lemon juice
- ½ tsp ground black pepper
- 1 garlic clove (minced)
- 1 kosher tsp salt
- 1 tsp freshly chopped tarragon

Directions:

1. Let the scallops dry using paper towels and drizzle all sides with salt and pepper to season
2. Place you're a cast iron pan in your grill and preheat the grill to 400°F with lid closed for 15 minutes.
3. Combine the butter and garlic in hot cast iron pan. Add the scallops and stir. Close grill lid and cook for 8 minutes. Flip the scallops and cook for an additional 7 minutes.
4. Remove the scallop from heat and let it rest for a few minutes.
5. Stir in the chopped tarragon. Serve and top with lemon juice.

Nutrition Info: Calories: 204 Cal Fat: 8.9 g Carbohydrates: 4 g   Protein: 25.6 g Fiber: 0.1 g

31. Enticing Mahi-mahi

Servings: 4

Cooking Time: 10 Minutes

Ingredients:

- 4 (6-oz.) mahi-mahi fillets
- 2 tbsp. olive oil
- Salt and freshly ground black pepper, to taste

Directions:

1. Set the temperature of Grill to 350 degrees F and preheat with closed lid for 15 minutes.
2. Coat fish fillets with olive oil and season with salt and black pepper evenly.
3. Place the fish fillets onto the grill and cook for about 5 minutes per side.
4. Remove the fish fillets from grill and serve hot.

Nutrition Info: Calories per serving: 195; Carbohydrates: 0g; Protein: 31.6g; Fat: 7g; Sugar: 0g; Sodium: 182mg; Fiber: 0g

32. Spot Prawn Skewers

Servings: 6

Cooking Time: 10 Minutes

Ingredients:

- 2 lb spot prawns
- 2 tbsp oil
- Salt and pepper to taste

Directions:

1. Preheat your to 400F.
2. Skewer your prawns with soaked skewers then generously sprinkle with oil, salt, and pepper.
3. Place the skewers on the grill and cook with the lid closed for 5 minutes on each side.
4. Remove the skewers and serve when hot.

Nutrition Info: Calories 221, Total fat 7g, Saturated fat 1g, Total carbs 2g, Net carbs 2g Protein 34g, Sugars 0g, Fiber 0g, Sodium 1481mg

33. Halibut

Servings: 4
Cooking Time: 30 Minutes

Ingredients:

- 1-pound fresh halibut filet (cut into 4 equal sizes)
- 1 tbsp fresh lemon juice
- 2 garlic cloves (minced)
- 2 tsp soy sauce
- ½ tsp ground black pepper
- ½ tsp onion powder
- 2 tbsp honey
- ½ tsp oregano
- 1 tsp dried basil
- 2 tbsp butter (melted)
- Maple syrup for serving

Directions:

1. Combine the lemon juice, honey, soy sauce, onion powder, oregano, dried basil, pepper and garlic.
2. Brush the halibut filets generously with the filet the mixture. Wrap the filets with aluminum foil and refrigerate for 4 hours.
3. Remove the filets from the refrigerator and let them sit for about 2 hours, or until they are at room temperature.
4. Activate your wood pellet grill on smoke, leaving the lid opened for 5 minutes or until fire starts.
5. The lid must not be opened for it to be preheated and reach 275°F 15 minutes, using fruit wood pellets.
6. Place the halibut filets directly on the grill grate and smoke for 30 minutes
7. Remove the filets from the grill and let them rest for 10 minutes.
8. Serve and top with maple syrup to taste

Nutrition Info: Calories: 180 Cal Fat: 6.3 g Carbohydrates: 10 g   Protein: 20.6 g Fiber: 0.3 g

34.　Octopus With Lemon And Oregano

Servings: 4

Cooking Time: 1 Hour And 30 Minutes

Ingredients:

- 3 lemons
- 3 pounds cleaned octopus, thawed if frozen
- 6 cloves garlic, peeled
- 4 sprigs fresh oregano
- 2 bay leaves
- Salt and pepper
- 3 tablespoons good-quality olive oil
- Minced fresh oregano for garnish

Directions:

1.　Halve one of the lemons. Put the octopus, garlic, oregano sprigs, bay leaves, a large pinch of salt, and lemon halves in a large pot with enough water to cover by a couple of inches. Bring to a boil, adjust the heat so the liquid bubbles gently but steadily, and cook, occasionally turning with tongs, until the octopus is tender 30 to 90 minutes. (Check with the tip of a sharp knife; it should go in smoothly.) Drain; discard the seasonings. (You can cover and refrigerate the octopus for up to 24 hours.)

2.　Start the coals or heat a gas grill for direct hot cooking. Make sure the grates are clean.

3.　Squeeze the juice 1 of the remaining lemons and whisk it with the oil and salt and pepper to taste. Cut the octopus into large serving pieces and toss with the oil mixture.

4.　Put the octopus on the grill directly over the fire. Cover the grill and cook until heated through and charred, 4 to 5 minutes per side. Cut the remaining lemon in wedges. Transfer the octopus to a platter, sprinkle with minced oregano, and serve with the lemon wedges.

Nutrition Info: Calories: 139 Fats: 1.8 g Cholesterol: 0 mg Carbohydrates: 3.7 g Fiber: 0 g Sugars: 0 g Proteins: 25.4 g

35. Citrus-smoked Trout

Servings: 6

Cooking Time: 1 To 2 Hours

Ingredients:

- 6 to 8 skin-on rainbow trout, cleaned and scaled
- 1 gallon orange juice
- ½ cup packed light brown sugar
- ¼ cup salt
- 1 tablespoon freshly ground black pepper
- Nonstick spray, oil, or butter, for greasing
- 1 tablespoon chopped fresh parsley
- 1 lemon, sliced

Directions:

1. Fillet the fish and pat dry with paper towels.
2. Pour the orange juice into a large container with a lid and stir in the brown sugar, salt, and pepper.
3. Place the trout in the brine, cover, and refrigerate for 1 hour.
4. Cover the grill grate with heavy-duty aluminum foil. Poke holes in the foil and spray with cooking spray (see Tip).
5. Supply your smoker with wood pellets and follow the manufacturer's specific start-up procedure. Preheat, with the lid closed, to 225°F.
6. Remove the trout from the brine and pat dry. Arrange the fish on the foil-covered grill grate, close the lid, and smoke for 1 hour 30 minutes to 2 hours, or until flaky.
7. Remove the fish from the heat. Serve garnished with the fresh parsley and lemon slices.

36.   Dijon-smoked Halibut

Servings: 6
Cooking Time: 2 Hours

Ingredients:

- 4 (6-ounce) halibut steaks
- ¼ cup extra-virgin olive oil
- 2 teaspoons kosher salt
- 1 teaspoon freshly ground black pepper
- ½ cup mayonnaise
- ½ cup sweet pickle relish
- ¼ cup finely chopped sweet onion
- ¼ cup chopped roasted red pepper
- ¼ cup finely chopped tomato
- ¼ cup finely chopped cucumber
- 2 tablespoons Dijon mustard
- 1 teaspoon minced garlic

Directions:

1.   Rub the halibut steaks with the olive oil and season on both sides with the salt and pepper. Transfer to a plate, cover with plastic wrap, and refrigerate for 4 hours.
2.   Supply your smoker with wood pellets and follow the manufacturer's specific start-up procedure. Preheat, with the lid closed, to 200°F.
3.   Remove the halibut from the refrigerator and rub with the mayonnaise.
4.   Put the fish directly on the grill grate, close the lid, and smoke for 2 hours, or until opaque and an instant-read thermometer inserted in the fish reads 140°F.
5.   While the fish is smoking, combine the pickle relish, onion, roasted red pepper, tomato, cucumber, Dijon mustard, and garlic in a medium bowl. Refrigerate the mustard relish until ready to serve.
6.   Serve the halibut steaks hot with the mustard relish.

37.   Lobster Tail

Servings: 2

Cooking Time: 15 Minutes

Ingredients:

- 10 oz lobster tail
- 1/4 tbsp old bay seasoning
- 1/4 tbsp Himalayan salt
- 2 tbsp butter, melted
- 1 tbsp fresh parsley, chopped

Directions:

1. Preheat your to 450F.
2. Slice the tail down the middle then season it with bay seasoning and salt.
3. Place the tails directly on the grill with the meat side down. Grill for 15 minutes or until the internal temperature reaches 140F.
4. Remove from the and drizzle with butter.
5. Serve when hot garnished with parsley.

Nutrition Info: Calories 305, Total fat 14g, Saturated fat 8g, Total carbs 5g, Net carbs 5g Protein 38g, Sugars 0g, Fiber 0g, Sodium 684mg

38. Blackened Salmon

Servings: 4

Cooking Time: 30 Minutes

Ingredients:

- 2 lb. salmon, fillet, scaled and deboned
- 2 tablespoons olive oil
- 4 tablespoons sweet dry rub
- 1 tablespoon cayenne pepper
- 2 cloves garlic, minced

Directions:

1. Turn on your wood pellet grill.
2. Set it to 350 degrees F.
3. Brush the salmon with the olive oil.
4. Sprinkle it with the dry rub, cayenne pepper, and garlic.
5. Grill for 5 minutes per side.

Nutrition Info: Calories: 460Fat: 23 gCholesterol: 140 mgCarbohydrates: 7 g Fiber: 5 g Sugars: 2 g Protein: 50 g

39.   Mango Shrimp

Servings: 4

Cooking Time: 15 Minutes

Ingredients:

- 1lb. shrimp, peeled and deveined but tail intact
- 2tablespoons olive oil
- Mango seasoning

Directions:

1. Turn on your wood pellet grill.
2. Preheat it to 425 degrees F.
3. Coat the shrimp with the oil and season with the mango seasoning.
4. Thread the shrimp into skewers.
5. Grill for 3 minutes per side.
6. Serving Suggestion: Garnish with chopped parsley.

Nutrition Info: Calories: 223.1 Fat: 4.3 g Cholesterol: 129.2 mg Carbohydrates: 29.2 g Fiber: 4.4 g Sugars: 15. 6g Protein: 19.5 g

40. Oysters In The Shell

Servings: 4

Cooking Time: 20 Minutes

Ingredients:

- 8 medium oysters, unopened, in the shell, rinsed and scrubbed
- 1 batch Lemon Butter Mop for Seafood

Directions:

1. Supply your smoker with wood pellets and follow the manufacturer's specific start-up procedure. Preheat the grill, with the lid closed, to 375°F.

2. Place the unopened oysters directly on the grill grate and grill for about 20 minutes, or until the oysters are done and their shells open.

3. Discard any oysters that do not open. Shuck the remaining oysters, transfer them to a bowl, and add the mop. Serve immediately.

41.   Smoked Shrimp

Servings: 6
Cooking Time: 10 Minutes
Ingredients:
- 1 lb tail-on shrimp, uncooked
- 1/2 tbsp onion powder
- 1/2 tbsp garlic powder
- 1/2 tbsp salt
- 4 tbsp teriyaki sauce
- 2 tbsp green onion, minced
- 4 tbsp sriracha mayo

Directions:
1. Peel the shrimp shells leaving the tail on then wash well and rise.
2. Drain well and pat dry with a paper towel.
3. Preheat your to 450F.
4. Season the shrimp with onion powder, garlic powder, and salt. Place the shrimp in the and cook for 6 minutes on each side.
5. Remove the shrimp from the and toss with teriyaki sauce then garnish with onions and mayo.

Nutrition Info: Calories 87, Total fat 0g, Saturated fat 0g, Total carbs 2g, Net carbs 2g Protein 16g, Sugars 0g, Fiber 0g, Sodium 1241mg

42.   Hot-smoked Salmon

Servings: 4

Cooking Time: 4 To 6 Hours

Ingredients:

- 1 (2-pound) half salmon fillet
- 1 batch Dill Seafood Rub

Directions:

1.   Supply your smoker with wood pellets and follow the manufacturer's specific start-up procedure. Preheat the grill, with the lid closed, to 180°F.

2.   Season the salmon all over with the rub. Using your hands, work the rub into the flesh.

3.   Place the salmon directly on the grill grate, skin-side down, and smoke until its internal temperature reaches 145°F. Remove the salmon from the grill and serve immediately.

43.   Bacon-wrapped Scallops

Servings: 4
Cooking Time: 30 Minutes

Ingredients:

- 12 scallops
- 12 bacon slices
- 3 tablespoons lemon juice
- Pepper to taste

Directions:

1. Turn on your wood pellet grill.
2. Set it to smoke.
3. Let it burn for 5 minutes while the lid is open.
4. Set it to 400 degrees F.
5. Wrap the scallops with bacon.
6. Secure with a toothpick.
7. Drizzle with the lemon juice and season with pepper.
8. Add the scallops to a baking tray.
9. Place the tray on the grill.
10. Grill for 20 minutes.
11. Serving Suggestion: Serve with sweet chili sauce.

Nutrition Info: Calories: 180.3 Fat: 8 g Cholesterol: 590.2 mg Carbohydrates: 3 g Fiber: 0 g Sugars: 0 g Protein: 22 g

44.   Fish Fillets With Pesto

Servings: 6

Cooking Time: 15 Minutes

Ingredients:

- 2 cups fresh basil
- 1 cup parsley, chopped
- 1/2 cup walnuts
- 1/2 cup olive oil
- 1 cup Parmesan cheese, grated
- Salt and pepper to taste
- 4 white fish fillets

Directions:

1. Preheat the wood pellet grill to high for 15 minutes while the lid is closed.
2. Add all the ingredients except fish to a food processor.
3. Pulse until smooth. Set aside.
4. Season fish with salt and pepper.
5. Grill for 6 to 7 minutes per side.
6. Serve with the pesto sauce.
7. Tips: You can also spread a little bit of the pesto on the fish before grilling.

45. Wood-fired Halibut

Servings: 4

Cooking Time: 20 Minutes

Ingredients:

- 1 pound halibut fillet
- 1 batch Dill Seafood Rub

Directions:

1. Supply your smoker with wood pellets and follow the manufacturer's specific start-up procedure. Preheat the grill, with the lid closed, to 325°F.

2. Sprinkle the halibut fillet on all sides with the rub. Using your hands, work the rub into the meat.

3. Place the halibut directly on the grill grate and grill until its internal temperature reaches 145°F. Remove the halibut from the grill and serve immediately.

46.   Wine Infused Salmon

Servings: 4
Cooking Time: 5 Hours

Ingredients:

- 2 C. low-sodium soy sauce
- 1 C. dry white wine
- 1 C. water
- ½ tsp. Tabasco sauce
- 1/3 C. sugar
- ¼ C. salt
- ½ tsp. garlic powder
- ½ tsp. onion powder
- Freshly ground black pepper, to taste
- 4 (6-oz.) salmon fillets

Directions:

1. In a large bowl, add all ingredients except salmon and stir until sugar is dissolved.
2. Add salmon fillets and coat with brine well.
3. Refrigerate, covered overnight.
4. Remove salmon from bowl and rinse under cold running water.
5. With paper towels, pat dry the salmon fillets.
6. Arrange a wire rack in a sheet pan.
7. Place the salmon fillets onto wire rack, skin side down and set aside to cool for about 1 hour.
8. Set the temperature of Grill to 165 degrees F and preheat with closed lid for 15 minutes, using charcoal.
9. Place the salmon fillets onto the grill, skin side down and cook for about 3-5 hours or until desired doneness.
10. Remove the salmon fillets from grill and serve hot.

Nutrition Info: Calories per serving: 377; Carbohydrates: 26.3g; Protein: 41.1g; Fat: 10.5g; Sugar: 25.1g; Sodium: 14000mg; Fiber: 0g

47. Grilled Shrimp Kabobs

Servings: 4

Cooking Time: 10 Minutes

Ingredients:

- 1 lb. colossal shrimp, peeled and deveined
- 2 tbsp. oil
- 1/2 tbsp. garlic salt
- 1/2 tbsp. salt
- 1/8 tbsp. pepper
- 6 skewers

Directions:

1. Preheat your to 375F.
2. Pat the shrimp dry with a paper towel.
3. In a mixing bowl, mix oil, garlic salt, salt, and pepper
4. Toss the shrimp in the mixture until well coated.
5. Skewer the shrimps and cook in the with the lid closed for 4 minutes.
6. Open the lid, flip the skewers and cook for another 4 minutes or until the shrimp is pink and the flesh is opaque.
7. Serve.

Nutrition Info: Calories 325, Total fat 0g, Saturated fat 0g, Total carbs 0g, Net carbs 0g Protein 20g, Sugars 0g, Fiber 0g, Sodium 120mg

48.   Buttered Crab Legs

Servings: 4

Cooking Time: 10 Minutes

Ingredients:

- 12 tablespoons butter
- 1 tablespoon parsley, chopped
- 1 tablespoon tarragon, chopped
- 1 tablespoon chives, chopped
- 1 tablespoon lemon juice
- 4 lb. king crab legs, split in the center

Directions:

1. Set the wood pellet grill to 375 degrees F.
2. Preheat it for 15 minutes while lid is closed.
3. In a pan over medium heat, simmer the butter, herbs and lemon juice for 2 minutes.
4. Place the crab legs on the grill.
5. Pour half of the sauce on top.
6. Grill for 10 minutes.
7. Serve with the reserved butter sauce.
8. Tips: You can also use shrimp for this recipe.

49. Barbecued Scallops

Servings: 4

Cooking Time: 10 Minutes

Ingredients:

- 1 pound large scallops
- 2 tablespoons olive oil
- 1 batch Dill Seafood Rub

Directions:

1. Supply your smoker with wood pellets and follow the manufacturer's specific start-up procedure. Preheat the grill, with the lid closed, to 375°F.

2. Coat the scallops all over with olive oil and season all sides with the rub.

3. Place the scallops directly on the grill grate and grill for 5 minutes per side. Remove the scallops from the grill and serve immediately.

50. Citrus Salmon

Servings: 6
Cooking Time: 30 Minutes

Ingredients:

- 2 (1-lb.) salmon fillets
- Salt and freshly ground black pepper, to taste
- 1 tbsp. seafood seasoning
- 2 lemons, sliced
- 2 limes, sliced

Directions:

1. Set the temperature of Grill to 225 degrees F and preheat with closed lid for 15 minutes.
2. Season the salmon fillets with salt, black pepper and seafood seasoning evenly.
3. Place the salmon fillets onto the grill and top each with lemon and lime slices evenly.
4. Cook for about 30 minutes.
5. Remove the salmon fillets from grill and serve hot.

Nutrition Info: Calories per serving: 327; Carbohydrates: 1g; Protein: 36.1g; Fat: 19.8g; Sugar: 0.2g; Sodium: 237mg; Fiber: 0.3g

51.   Togarashi Smoked Salmon

Servings: 10
Cooking Time: 20 Hours 15 Minutes

Ingredients:

- Salmon filet - 2 large
- Togarashi for seasoning
- For Brine:
- Brown sugar - 1 cup
- Water - 4 cups
- Kosher salt - ⅓ cup

Directions:

1. Remove all the thorns from the fish filet.
2. Mix all the brine ingredients until the brown sugar is dissolved completely.
3. Put the mix in a big bowl and add the filet to it.
4. Leave the bowl to refrigerate for 16 hours.
5. After 16 hours, remove the salmon from this mix. Wash and dry it.
6. Place the salmon in the refrigerator for another 2-4 hours. (This step is important. DO NOT SKIP IT.)
7. Season your salmon filet with Togarashi.
8. Start the wood pellet grill with the 'smoke' option and place the salmon on it.
9. Smoke for 4 hours.
10. Make sure the temperature does not go above 180 degrees or below 130 degrees.
11. Remove from the grill and serve it warm with a side dish of your choice.

Nutrition Info: Carbohydrates: 19 g Protein: 10 g Fat: 6 g Sodium: 3772 mg Cholesterol: 29 mg

52. Crab Stuffed Lingcod

Servings: 6
Cooking Time: 30 Minutes

Ingredients:

- Lemon cream sauce
- 4 garlic cloves
- 1 shallot
- 1 leek
- 2 tbsp olive oil
- 1 tbsp salt
- 1/4 tbsp black pepper
- 3 tbsp butter
- 1/4 cup white wine
- 1 cup whipping cream
- 2 tbsp lemon juice
- 1 tbsp lemon zest
- Crab mix
- 1 lb crab meat
- 1/3 cup mayo
- 1/3 cup sour cream
- 1/3 cup lemon cream sauce
- 1/4 green onion, chopped
- 1/4 tbsp black pepper
- 1/2 tbsp old bay seasoning
- Fish
- 2 lb lingcod
- 1 tbsp olive oil
- 1 tbsp salt
- 1 tbsp paprika
- 1 tbsp green onion, chopped
- 1 tbsp Italian parsley

Directions:

1. Lemon cream sauce
2. Chop garlic, shallot, and leeks then add to a saucepan with oil, salt, pepper, and butter.
3. Saute over medium heat until the shallot is translucent.
4. Deglaze with white wine then add whipping cream. Bring the sauce to boil, reduce heat and simmer for 3 minutes.
5. Remove from heat and add lemon juice and lemon zest. Transfer the sauce to a blender and blend until smooth.
6. Set aside 1/3 cup for the crab mix
7. Crab mix
8. Add all the ingredients in a mixing bowl and mix thoroughly until well combined.
9. Set aside
10. Fish
11. Fire up your to high heat then slice the fish into 6-ounce portions.
12. Lay the fish on its side on a cutting board and slice it 3/4 way through the middle leaving a 1/2 inch on each end so as to have a nice pouch.
13. Rub the oil into the fish then place them on a baking sheet. Sprinkle with salt.
14. Stuff crab mix into each fish then sprinkle paprika and place it on the grill.
15. Cook for 15 minutes or more if the fillets are more than 2 inches thick.
16. Remove the fish and transfer to serving platters. Pour the remaining lemon cream sauce on each fish and garnish with onions and parsley.

Nutrition Info: Calories 476, Total fat 33g, Saturated fat 14g, Total carbs 6g, Net carbs 5g Protein 38g, Sugars 3g, Fiber 1g, Sodium 1032mg

POULTRY RECIPES

53. Special Occasion's Dinner Cornish Hen

Servings: 4

Cooking Time: 1 Hour

Ingredients:

- 4 Cornish game hens
- 4 fresh rosemary sprigs
- 4 tbsp. butter, melted
- 4 tsp. chicken rub

Directions:

1. Set the temperature of Grill to 375 degrees F and preheat with closed lid for 15 minutes.
2. With paper towels, pat dry the hens.
3. Tuck the wings behind the backs and with kitchen strings, tie the legs together.
4. Coat the outside of each hen with melted butter and sprinkle with rub evenly.
5. Stuff the cavity of each hen with a rosemary sprig.
6. Place the hens onto the grill and cook for about 50-60 minutes.
7. Remove the hens from grill and place onto a platter for about 10 minutes.
8. Cut each hen into desired-sized pieces and serve.

Nutrition Info: Calories per serving: 430; Carbohydrates: 2.1g; Protein: 25.4g; Fat: 33g; Sugar: 0g; Sodium: 331mg; Fiber: 0.7g

54. Smo-fried Chicken

Servings: 4 To 6
Cooking Time: 55 Minutes

Ingredients:

- 1 egg, beaten
- ½ cup milk
- 1 cup all-purpose flour
- 2 tablespoons salt
- 1 tablespoon freshly ground black pepper
- 2 teaspoons freshly ground white pepper
- 2 teaspoons cayenne pepper
- 2 teaspoons garlic powder
- 2 teaspoons onion powder
- 1 teaspoon smoked paprika
- 8 tablespoons (1 stick) unsalted butter, melted
- 1 whole chicken, cut up into pieces

Directions:

1. Supply your smoker with wood pellets and follow the manufacturer's specific start-up procedure. Preheat, with the lid closed, to 375°F.
2. In a medium bowl, combine the beaten egg with the milk and set aside.
3. In a separate medium bowl, stir together the flour, salt, black pepper, white pepper, cayenne, garlic powder, onion powder, and smoked paprika.
4. Line the bottom and sides of a high-sided metal baking pan with aluminum foil to ease cleanup.
5. Pour the melted butter into the prepared pan.
6. Dip the chicken pieces one at a time in the egg mixture, and then coat well with the seasoned flour. Transfer to the baking pan.
7. Smoke the chicken in the pan of butter ("smo-fry") on the grill, with the lid closed, for 25 minutes, then reduce the heat to 325°F and turn the chicken pieces over.
8. Continue smoking with the lid closed for about 30 minutes, or until a meat thermometer inserted in the thickest part of each chicken piece reads 165°F.
9. Serve immediately.

55. Smoked And Fried Chicken Wings

Servings: 6

Cooking Time: 2 Hours

Ingredients:

- 3 pounds chicken wings
- 1 tbsp Goya adobo all-purpose seasoning
- Sauce of your choice

Directions:

1. Fire up your wood pellet grill and set it to smoke.
2. Meanwhile, coat the chicken wings with adobo all-purpose seasoning. Place the chicken on the grill and smoke for 2 hours.
3. Remove the wings from the grill.
4. Preheat oil to 375°F in a frying pan. Drop the wings in batches and let fry for 5 minutes or until the skin is crispy.
5. Drain the oil and proceed with drizzling preferred sauce
6. Drain oil and drizzle preferred sauce
7. Enjoy.

Nutrition Info: Calories: 755 Cal Fat: 55 g Carbohydrates: 24 g   Protein: 39 g Fiber: 1 g

56. Maple And Bacon Chicken

Servings: 7

Cooking Time: 1 And ½ Hours

Ingredients:

- 4 boneless and skinless chicken breast
- Salt as needed
- Fresh pepper
- 12 slices bacon, uncooked
- 1cup maple syrup
- ½ cup melted butter
- 1teaspoon liquid smoke

Directions:

1. Preheat your smoker to 250 degrees Fahrenheit
2. Season the chicken with pepper and salt
3. Wrap the breast with 3 bacon slices and cover the entire surface
4. Secure the bacon with toothpicks
5. Take a medium-sized bowl and stir in maple syrup, butter, liquid smoke, and mix well
6. Reserve 1/3rd of this mixture for later use
7. Submerge the chicken breast into the butter mix and coat them well
8. Place a pan in your smoker and transfer the chicken to your smoker
9. Smoker for 1 to 1 and a ½ hours
10. Brush the chicken with reserved butter and smoke for 30 minutes more until the internal temperature reaches 165 degrees Fahrenheit
11. Enjoy!

Nutrition Info: Calories: 458 Fats: 20g Carbs: 65g Fiber: 1g

57.   Barbecue Chicken Wings

Servings: 4
Cooking Time: 15 Minutes

Ingredients:

- Fresh chicken wings
- Salt to taste
- Pepper to taste
- Garlic powder
- Onion powder
- Cayenne
- Paprika
- Seasoning salt
- Bbq sauce to taste

Directions:

1. Preheat the wood pellet grill to low.
2. In a mixing bowl, mix all the seasoning ingredients then toss the chicken wings until well coated.
3. Place the wings on the grill and cook for 20 minutes or until the wings are fully cooked.
4. Let rest to cool for 5 minutes then toss with bbq sauce.
5. Serve with orzo and salad. Enjoy.

Nutrition Info: Calories 311, Total fat 22g, Saturated fat 4g, Total carbs 22g, Net carbs 19g, Protein 22g, Sugar 12g, Fiber 3g, Sodium: 1400mg

58.   Succulent Duck Breast

Servings: 4
Cooking Time: 10 Minutes

Ingredients:

- 4 (6-oz.) boneless duck breasts
- 2 tbsp. chicken rub

Directions:

1. Set the temperature of Grill to 275 degrees F and preheat with closed lid for 15 minutes.
2. With a sharp knife, score the skin of the duck into ¼-inch diamond pattern.
3. Season the duck breast with rub evenly.
4. Place the duck breasts onto the grill, meat side down and cook for about 10 minutes.
5. Now, set the temperature of Grill to 400 degrees F.
6. Now, arrange the breasts, skin side down and cook for about 10 minutes, flipping once halfway through.
7. Remove from the grill and serve.

Nutrition Info: Calories per serving: 231; Carbohydrates: 1.5g; Protein: 37.4g; Fat: 6.8g; Sugar: 0g; Sodium: 233mg; Fiber: 0g

59. Grilled Buffalo Chicken

Servings: 6
Cooking Time: 20 Minutes

Ingredients:

- 5 chicken breasts, boneless and skinless
- 2 tbsp homemade BBQ rub
- 1 cup homemade Cholula Buffalo sauce

Directions:

1. Preheat the to 400F.
2. Slice the chicken breast lengthwise into strips. Season the slices with BBQ rub.
3. Place the chicken slices on the grill and paint both sides with buffalo sauce.
4. Cook for 4 minutes with the lid closed. Flip the breasts, paint again with sauce and cook until the internal temperature reaches 165F.
5. Remove the chicken from the and serve when warm.

Nutrition Info: Calories 176, Total fat 4g, Saturated fat 1g, Total carbs 1g, Net carbs 1g Protein 32g, Sugars 1g, Fiber 0g, Sodium 631mg

60.   Wood Pellet Smoked Spatchcock Turkey

Servings: 6

Cooking Time: 1 Hour And 45 Minutes

Ingredients:

- 1 whole turkey
- 1/2 cup oil
- 1/4 cup chicken rub
- 1 tbsp onion powder
- 1 tbsp garlic powder
- 1 tbsp rubbed sage

Directions:

1. Preheat your wood pellet grill to high.
2. Meanwhile, place the turkey on a platter with the breast side down then cut on either side of the backbone to remove the spine.
3. Flip the turkey and season on both sides then place it on the preheated grill or on a pan if you want to catch the drippings. Grill on high for 30 minutes, reduce the temperature to 325°F, and grill for 45 more minutes or until the internal temperature reaches 165°F Remove from the grill and let rest for 20 minutes before slicing and serving. Enjoy.

Nutrition Info: Calories: 156 Cal Fat: 16 g Carbohydrates: 1 g   Protein: 2 g Fiber: 0 g

61. Glazed Chicken Thighs

Servings: 4
Cooking Time: 30 Minutes

Ingredients:

- 2 garlic cloves, minced
- ¼ C. honey
- 2 tbsp. soy sauce
- ¼ tsp. red pepper flakes, crushed
- 4 (5-oz.) skinless, boneless chicken thighs
- 2 tbsp. olive oil
- 2 tsp. sweet rub
- ¼ tsp. red chili powder
- Freshly ground black pepper, to taste

Directions:

1. Set the temperature of Grill to 400 degrees F and preheat with closed lid for 15 minutes.
2. In a small bowl, add garlic, honey, soy sauce and red pepper flakes and with a wire whisk, beat until well combined.
3. Coat chicken thighs with oil and season with sweet rub, chili powder and black pepper generously.
4. Arrange the chicken drumsticks onto the grill and cook for about 15 minutes per side.
5. In the last 4-5 minutes of cooking, coat the thighs with garlic mixture.
6. Serve immediately.

Nutrition Info: Calories per serving: 309; Carbohydrates: 18.7g; Protein: 32.3g; Fat: 12.1g; Sugar: 17.6g; Sodium: 504mg; Fiber: 0.2g

62.   Lemon Chicken

Servings: 6

Cooking Time: 10 Minutes

Ingredients:

- 2 teaspoons honey
- 1 tablespoon lemon juice
- 1 teaspoon lemon zest
- 1 clove garlic, coarsely chopped
- 2 sprigs thyme
- Salt and pepper to taste
- ½ cup olive oil
- 6 chicken breast fillets

Directions:

1. Mix the honey, lemon juice, lemon zest, garlic, thyme, salt and pepper in a bowl.
2. Gradually add olive oil to the mixture.
3. Soak the chicken fillets in the mixture.
4. Cover and refrigerate for 4 hours.
5. Preheat the wood pellet grill to 400 degrees F for 15 minutes while the lid is closed.
6. Grill the chicken for 5 minutes per side.
7. Tips: You can also make additional marinade to be used for basting during grill time.

63. Turkey Meatballs

Servings: 8
Cooking Time: 40 Minutes

Ingredients:

- 1 1/4 lb. ground turkey
- 1/2 cup breadcrumbs
- 1 egg, beaten
- 1/4 cup milk
- 1 teaspoon onion powder
- 1/4 cup Worcestershire sauce
- Pinch garlic salt
- Salt and pepper to taste
- 1 cup cranberry jam
- 1/2 cup orange marmalade
- 1/2 cup chicken broth

Directions:

1. In a large bowl, mix the ground turkey, breadcrumbs, egg, milk, onion powder, Worcestershire sauce, garlic salt, salt and pepper.
2. Form meatballs from the mixture.
3. Preheat the wood pellet grill to 350 degrees F for 15 minutes while the lid is closed.
4. Add the turkey meatballs to a baking pan.
5. Place the baking pan on the grill.
6. Cook for 20 minutes.
7. In a pan over medium heat, simmer the rest of the ingredients for 10 minutes.
8. Add the grilled meatballs to the pan.
9. Coat with the mixture.
10. Cook for 10 minutes.
11. Tips: You can add chili powder to the meatball mixture if you want spicy flavor.

64. Serrano Chicken Wings

Servings: 4

Cooking Time: 40 Minutes

Ingredients:

- 4 lb. chicken wings
- 2 cups beer
- 2 teaspoons crushed red pepper
- Cajun seasoning powder
- 1 lb. Serrano chili peppers
- 1 teaspoon fresh basil
- 1 teaspoon dried oregano
- 4 cloves garlic
- 1 cup vinegar
- Salt and pepper to taste

Directions:

1. Soak the chicken wings in beer.
2. Sprinkle with crushed red pepper.
3. Cover and refrigerate for 12 hours.
4. Remove chicken from brine.
5. Season with Cajun seasoning.
6. Preheat your wood pellet grill to 325 degrees F for 15 minutes while the lid is closed.
7. Add the chicken wings and Serrano chili peppers on the grill.
8. Grill for 5 minutes per side.
9. Remove chili peppers and place in a food processor.
10. Grill the chicken for another 20 minutes.
11. Add the rest of the ingredients to the food processor.
12. Pulse until smooth.
13. Dip the chicken wings in the sauce.
14. Grill for 5 minutes and serve.
15. Tips: You can also use prepared pepper sauce to save time.

65.   Bacon-wrapped Chicken Tenders

Servings: 6

Cooking Time: 30 Minutes

Ingredients:

- 1-pound chicken tenders
- 10 strips bacon
- 1/2 tbsp Italian seasoning
- 1/2 tbsp black pepper
- 1/2 tbsp salt
- 1 tbsp paprika
- 1 tbsp onion powder
- 1 tbsp garlic powder
- 1/3 cup light brown sugar
- 1 tbsp chili powder

Directions:

1. Preheat your wood pellet smoker to 350°F.
2. Mix seasonings
3. Sprinkle the mixture on all sides of chicken tenders
4. Wrap each chicken tender with a strip of bacon
5. Mix sugar and chili then sprinkle the mixture on the bacon-wrapped chicken.
6. Place them on the smoker and smoker for 30 minutes with the lid closed or until the chicken is cooked.
7. Serve and enjoy.

Nutrition Info: Calories: 206 Cal Fat: 7.9 g Carbohydrates: 1.5 g   Protein: 30.3 g Fiber: 0 g

66.   Beer Can–smoked Chicken

Servings: 3 To 4
Cooking Time: 3 To 4 Hours
Ingredients:
- 8 tablespoons (1 stick) unsalted butter, melted
- ½ cup apple cider vinegar
- ½ cup Cajun seasoning, divided
- 1 teaspoon garlic powder
- 1 teaspoon onion powder
- 1 (4-pound) whole chicken, giblets removed
- Extra-virgin olive oil, for rubbing
- 1 (12-ounce) can beer
- 1 cup apple juice
- ½ cup extra-virgin olive oil

Directions:
1.   In a small bowl, whisk together the butter, vinegar, ¼ cup of Cajun seasoning, garlic powder, and onion powder.
2.   Use a meat-injecting syringe to inject the liquid into various spots in the chicken. Inject about half of the mixture into the breasts and the other half throughout the rest of the chicken.
3.   Rub the chicken all over with olive oil and apply the remaining ¼ cup of Cajun seasoning, being sure to rub under the skin as well.
4.   Drink or discard half the beer and place the opened beer can on a stable surface.
5.   Place the bird's cavity on top of the can and position the chicken so it will sit up by itself. Prop the legs forward to make the bird more stable, or buy an inexpensive, specially made stand to hold the beer can and chicken in place.
6.   Supply your smoker with wood pellets and follow the manufacturer's specific start-up procedure. Preheat, with the lid closed, to 250°F.
7.   In a clean 12-ounce spray bottle, combine the apple juice and olive oil. Cover and shake the mop sauce well before each use.
8.   Carefully put the chicken on the grill. Close the lid and smoke the chicken for 3 to 4 hours, spraying with the mop sauce every hour, until golden brown and a meat thermometer inserted in the thickest part of the thigh reads 165°F. Keep a piece of aluminum foil handy to loosely cover the chicken if the skin begins to brown too quickly.
9.   Let the meat rest for 5 minutes before carving.

67.   Smoked Lemon Chicken Breasts

Servings: 6
Cooking Time: 30 Minutes
Ingredients:
- 2 lemons, zested and juiced
- 1 clove of garlic, minced
- 2 teaspoons honey
- 2 teaspoons salt
- 1 teaspoon ground black pepper
- 2 sprigs fresh thyme
- ½ cup olive oil
- 6 boneless chicken breasts

Directions:
1. Place all ingredients in a bowl. Massage the chicken breasts so that it is coated with the marinade.
2. Place in the fridge to marinate for at least 4 hours.
3. Fire the Grill to 350F. Use apple wood pellets. Close the grill lid and preheat for 15 minutes.
4. Place the chicken breasts on the grill grate and cook for 15 minutes on both sides.
5. Serve immediately or drizzle with lemon juice.

Nutrition Info: Calories per serving: 671 ; Protein: 60.6 g; Carbs: 3.5 g; Fat: 44.9g Sugar: 2.3g

68.   Herb Roasted Turkey

Servings: 12
Cooking Time: 3 Hours And 30 Minutes

Ingredients:

- 14 pounds turkey, cleaned
- 2 tablespoons chopped mixed herbs
- Pork and poultry rub as needed
- 1/4 teaspoon ground black pepper
- 3 tablespoons butter, unsalted, melted
- 8 tablespoons butter, unsalted, softened
- 2 cups chicken broth

Directions:

1.   Clean the turkey by removing the giblets, wash it inside out, pat dry with paper towels, then place it on a roasting pan and tuck the turkey wings by tiring with butcher's string.

2.   Switch on the grill, fill the grill hopper with hickory flavored wood pellets, power the grill on by using the control panel, select 'smoke' on the temperature dial, or set the temperature to 325 degrees F and let it preheat for a minimum of 15 minutes.

3.   Meanwhile, prepared herb butter and for this, take a small bowl, place the softened butter in it, add black pepper and mixed herbs and beat until fluffy.

4.   Place some of the prepared herb butter underneath the skin of turkey by using a handle of a wooden spoon, and massage the skin to distribute butter evenly.

5.   Then rub the exterior of the turkey with melted butter, season with pork and poultry rub, and pour the broth in the roasting pan.

6.   When the grill has preheated, open the lid, place roasting pan containing turkey on the grill grate, shut the grill and smoke for 3 hours and 30 minutes until the internal temperature reaches 165 degrees F and the top has turned golden brown.

7.   When done, transfer turkey to a cutting board, let it rest for 30 minutes, then carve it into slices and serve.

Nutrition Info: Calories: 154.6 Cal ;Fat: 3.1 g ;Carbs: 8.4 g ;Protein: 28.8 g ;Fiber: 0.4 g

69. Hickory Smoked Chicken

Servings: 4

Cooking Time: 30 Minutes

Ingredients:

- 4 chicken breasts
- ¼ cup olive oil
- 1 teaspoon pressed garlic
- 1 tablespoon Worcestershire sauce
- Kirkland Sweet Mesquite Seasoning as needed
- 1 button Honey Bourbon Sauce

Directions:

1. Place all ingredients in a bowl except for the Bourbon sauce. Massage the chicken until all parts are coated with the seasoning.
2. Allow to marinate in the fridge for 4 hours.
3. Once ready to cook, fire the Grill to 350F. Use Hickory wood pellets and close the lid. Preheat for 15 minutes.
4. Place the chicken directly into the grill grate and cook for 30 minutes. Flip the chicken halfway through the cooking time.
5. Five minutes before the cooking time ends, brush all surfaces of the chicken with the Honey Bourbon Sauce.
6. Serve immediately.

Nutrition Info: Calories per serving: 622; Protein: 60.5g; Carbs: 1.1g; Fat: 40.3g Sugar: 0.4g

70.   Sheet Pan Chicken Fajitas

Servings: 10
Cooking Time: 10 Minutes
Ingredients:
- 2 lb chicken breast
- 1 onion, sliced
- 1 red bell pepper, seeded and sliced
- 1 orange-red bell pepper, seeded and sliced
- 1 tbsp salt
- 1/2 tbsp onion powder
- 1/2 tbsp granulated garlic
- 2 tbsp Spiceologist Chile Margarita Seasoning
- 2 tbsp oil

Directions:
1. Preheat the to 450F and line a baking sheet with parchment paper.
2. In a mixing bowl, combine seasonings and oil then toss with the peppers and chicken.
3. Place the baking sheet in the and let heat for 10 minutes with the lid closed.
4. Open the lid and place the veggies and the chicken in a single layer. Close the lid and cook for 10 minutes or until the chicken is no longer pink.
5. Serve with warm tortillas and top with your favorite toppings.

Nutrition Info: Calories 211, Total fat 6g, Saturated fat 1g, Total carbs 5g, Net carbs 4g
Protein 29g, Sugars 4g, Fiber 1g, Sodium 360mg

71.   Teriyaki Wings

Servings: 8
Cooking Time: 50 Minutes

Ingredients:

- 2 ½ pounds large chicken wings
- 1 tablespoon toasted sesame seeds
- For the Marinade:
- 2 scallions, sliced
- 2 tablespoons grated ginger
- ½ teaspoon minced garlic
- 1/4 cup brown sugar
- 1/2 cup soy sauce
- 2 tablespoon rice wine vinegar
- 2 teaspoons sesame oil
- 1/4 cup water

Directions:

1.   Prepare the chicken wings and for this, remove tips from the wings, cut each chicken wing through the joint into three pieces, and then place in a large plastic bag.
2.   Prepare the sauce and for this, take a small saucepan, place it over medium-high heat, add all of its ingredients in it, stir until mixed, and bring it to a boil.
3.   Then switch heat to medium level, simmer the sauce for 10 minutes, and when done, cool the sauce completely.
4.   Pour the sauce over chicken wings, seal the bag, turn it upside down to coat chicken wings with the sauce and let it marinate for a minimum of 8 hours in the refrigerator.
5.   When ready to cook, switch on the grill, fill the grill hopper with maple-flavored wood pellets, power the grill on by using the control panel, select 'smoke' on the temperature dial, or set the temperature to 350 degrees F and let it preheat for a minimum of 15 minutes.
6.   Meanwhile,
7.   When the grill has preheated, open the lid, place chicken wings on the grill grate, shut the grill and smoke for 50 minutes until crispy and meat is no longer pink, turning halfway.
8.   When done, transfer chicken wings to a dish, sprinkle with sesame seeds and then serve.

Nutrition Info: Calories: 150 Cal ;Fat: 7.5 g ;Carbs: 6 g ;Protein: 12 g ;Fiber: 1 g

72.   **Wood Pellet Chicken Breasts**

Servings: 6
Cooking Time: 15 Minutes

Ingredients:

- 3 chicken breasts
- 1 tbsp avocado oil
- 1/4 tbsp garlic powder
- 1/4 tbsp onion powder
- 3/4 tbsp salt
- 1/4 tbsp pepper

Directions:

1. Preheat your pellet to 375°F.
2. Half the chicken breasts lengthwise then coat with avocado oil.
3. With the spices, drizzle it on all sides to season
4. Drizzle spices to season the chicken. Put the chicken on top of the grill and begin to cook until its internal temperature approaches 165 degrees Fahrenheit. Put the chicken on top of the grill and begin to cook until it rises to a temperature of 165 degrees Fahrenheit
5. Serve and enjoy.

Nutrition Info: Calories: 120 Cal Fat: 4 g Carbohydrates: 0 g   Protein: 19 g Fiber: 0 g

73.   Spatchcocked Turkey

Servings: 10 To 14
Cooking Time: 2 Hours

Ingredients:

- 1 whole turkey
- 2 tablespoons olive oil
- 1 batch Chicken Rub

Directions:

1.   Supply your smoker with wood pellets and follow the manufacturer's specific start-up procedure. Preheat the grill, with the lid closed, to 350°F.

2.   To remove the turkey's backbone, place the turkey on a work surface, on its breast. Using kitchen shears, cut along one side of the turkey's backbone and then the other. Pull out the bone.

3.   Once the backbone is removed, turn the turkey breast-side up and flatten it.

4.   Coat the turkey with olive oil and season it on both sides with the rub. Using your hands, work the rub into the meat and skin.

5.   Place the turkey directly on the grill grate, breast-side up, and cook until its internal temperature reaches 170°F.

6.   Remove the turkey from the grill and let it rest for 10 minutes, before carving and serving.

74. Applewood-smoked Whole Turkey

Servings: 6 To 8

Cooking Time: 5 To 6 Hours

Ingredients:

- 1 (10- to 12-pound) turkey, giblets removed
- Extra-virgin olive oil, for rubbing
- ¼ cup poultry seasoning
- 8 tablespoons (1 stick) unsalted butter, melted
- ½ cup apple juice
- 2 teaspoons dried sage
- 2 teaspoons dried thyme

Directions:

1. Supply your smoker with wood pellets and follow the manufacturer's specific start-up procedure. Preheat, with the lid closed, to 250°F.

2. Rub the turkey with oil and season with the poultry seasoning inside and out, getting under the skin.

3. In a bowl, combine the melted butter, apple juice, sage, and thyme to use for basting.

4. Put the turkey in a roasting pan, place on the grill, close the lid, and grill for 5 to 6 hours, basting every hour, until the skin is brown and crispy, or until a meat thermometer inserted in the thickest part of the thigh reads 165°F.

5. Let the bird rest for 15 to 20 minutes before carving.

75.   Bbq Half Chickens

Servings: 4
Cooking Time: 75 Minutes

Ingredients:

- 3.5-pound whole chicken, cleaned, halved
- Summer rub as needed
- Apricot BBQ sauce as needed

Directions:

1.   Switch on the grill, fill the grill hopper with apple-flavored wood pellets, power the grill on by using the control panel, select 'smoke' on the temperature dial, or set the temperature to 375 degrees F and let it preheat for a minimum of 15 minutes.

2.   Meanwhile, cut chicken in half along with backbone and then season with summer rub.

3.   When the grill has preheated, open the lid, place chicken halves on the grill grate skin-side up, shut the grill, change the smoking temperature to 225 degrees F, and smoke for 1 hour and 30 minutes until the internal temperature reaches 160 degrees F.

4.   Then brush chicken generously with apricot sauce and continue grilling for 10 minutes until glazed.

5.   When done, transfer chicken to cutting to a dish, let it rest for 5 minutes, and then serve.

Nutrition Info: Calories: 435 Cal ;Fat: 20 g ;Carbs: 20 g ;Protein: 42 g ;Fiber: 1 g

76. Lemon Chicken Breasts

Servings: 6

Cooking Time: 40 Minutes

Ingredients:

- 1 clove of garlic, minced
- 2 teaspoons honey
- 2 teaspoons salt
- 1 teaspoon black pepper, ground
- 2 sprigs fresh thyme leaves
- 1 lemon, zested and juiced
- ½ cup olive oil
- 6 boneless chicken breasts

Directions:

1. Make the marinade by combining the garlic, honey, salt, pepper, thyme, lemon zest, and juice in a bowl. Whisk until well-combined.

2. Place the chicken into the marinade and mix with hands to coat the meat with the marinade. Refrigerate for 4 hours.

3. When ready to grill, fire the Grill to 400F. Close the lid and preheat for 10 minutes.

4. Drain the chicken and discard the marinade.

5. Arrange the chicken breasts directly on to the grill grate and cook for 40 minutes or until the internal temperature of the thickest part of the chicken reaches to 165F.

6. Drizzle with more lemon juice before serving.

Nutrition Info: Calories per serving: 669; Protein: 60.6g; Carbs: 3g; Fat: 44.9g Sugar: 2.1g

Servings: 6

Cooking Time: 40 Minutes

Ingredients:

- 3 tablespoons chili powder
- 2 tablespoons extra virgin olive oil
- 2 teaspoons lime zest
- 3 tablespoons lime juice
- 1 tablespoon garlic, minced
- 1 teaspoon ground coriander
- 1 teaspoon ground cumin
- 1 teaspoon dried oregano
- 1 ½ teaspoons salt
- 1 teaspoon ground black pepper
- A pinch of cinnamon
- 1 chicken, spatchcocked

Directions:

1.   In a bowl, place the chili powder, olive oil, lime zest, juice, garlic, coriander, cumin, oregano, salt, pepper, cinnamon, and cinnamon in a bowl. Mix to form a paste.

2.   Place the chicken cut-side down on a chopping board and flatten using the heel of your hand. Carefully, break the breastbone to flatten the chicken.

3.   Generously rub the spices all over the chicken and make sure to massage the chicken with the spice rub. Place in a baking dish and refrigerate for 24 hours in the fridge.

4.   When ready to cook, fire the Grill to 400F. Use maple wood pellets. Close the grill lid and preheat for 15 minutes.

5.   Place the chicken breastbone-side down on the grill grate and cook for 40 minutes or until a thermometer inserted in the thickest part reads at 165F.

6.   Make sure to flip the chicken halfway through the cooking time.

7.   Once cooked, transfer to a plate and allow to rest before carving the chicken.

Nutrition Info: Calories per serving: 213; Protein: 33.1g; Carbs: 3.8g; Fat: 7g Sugar: 0.5g

78.   Wood Pellet Chicken Wings With Spicy Miso

Servings: 6

Cooking Time: 25 Minutes

Ingredients:

- 2-pound chicken wings
- 3/4 cup soy
- 1/2 cup pineapple juice
- 1 tbsp sriracha
- 1/8 cup miso
- 1/8 cup gochujang
- 1/2 cup water
- 1/2 cup oil
- Togarashi

Directions:

1. Mix all ingredients then toss the chicken wings until well coated. Refrigerate for 12 minutes.

2. Preheat your wood pellet grill to 375°F. Place the chicken wings on the grill grates and close the lid. Cook until the internal temperature reaches 165°F. Remove the wings from the grill and sprinkle with togarashi. Serve when hot and enjoy.

Nutrition Info: Calories: 704 Cal Fat: 56 g Carbohydrates: 24 g   Protein: 27 g Fiber: 1 g

BEEF, PORK & LAMB RECIPES

79.   Kalbi Beef Short Ribs

Servings: 6
Cooking Time: 6 Hours
Ingredients:
- 1/2 cup soy sauce
- 1/2 cup brown sugar
- 1/8 cup rice wine
- 2 tbsp minced garlic
- 1 tbsp sesame oil
- 1/8 cup onion, finely grated
- 2-1/2 pound beef short ribs, thinly sliced

Directions:
1.   Mix soy sauce, sugar, rice wine, garlic, sesame oil and onion in a medium mixing bowl.
2.   Add the beef in the bowl and cover it in the marinade. Cover the bowl with a plastic wrap and refrigerate for 6 hours.
3.   Heat your to high and ensure the grill is well heated.
4.   Place on grill and close the lid ensuring you don't lose any heat.
5.   Cook for 4 minutes, flip, and cook for 4 more minutes on the other side.
6.   Remove the meat and serve with rice and veggies of choice. Enjoy.
Nutrition Info: Calories: 355 Cal Fat: 10 g Carbohydrates: 22 g   Protein: 28 g Fiber: 0 g

80. Elegant Lamb Chops

Servings: 4
Cooking Time: 30 Minutes

Ingredients:

- 4 lamb shoulder chops
- 4 C. buttermilk
- 1 C. cold water
- ¼ C. kosher salt
- 2 tbsp. olive oil
- 1 tbsp. Texas-style rub

Directions:

1. In a large bowl, add buttermilk, water and salt and stir until salt is dissolved.
2. Add chops and coat with mixture evenly.
3. Refrigerate for at least 4 hours.
4. Remove the chops from bowl and rinse under cold running water.
5. Coat the chops with olive oil and then sprinkle with rub evenly.
6. Set the temperature of Grill to 240 degrees F and preheat with closed lid for 15 minutes, using charcoal.
7. Arrange the chops onto grill and cook for about 25-30 minutes or until desired doneness.
8. Meanwhile, preheat the broiler of oven. Grease a broiler pan.
9. Remove the chops from grill and place onto the prepared broiler pan.
10. Transfer the broiler pan into the oven and broil for about 3-5 minutes or until browned.
11. Remove the chops from oven and serve hot.

Nutrition Info: Calories per serving: 414; Carbohydrates: 11.7g; Protein: 5.6g; Fat: 22.7g; Sugar: 11.7g; Sodium: 7000mg; Fiber: 0g

81. Simple Smoked Baby Backs

Servings: 4 To 8

Cooking Time: 4 To 6 Hours

Ingredients:

- 2 (2- or 3-pound) racks baby back ribs
- 2 tablespoons yellow mustard
- 1 batch Pork Rub

Directions:

1. Supply your smoker with wood pellets and follow the manufacturer's specific start-up procedure. Preheat the grill, with the lid closed, to 225°F.

2. Remove the membrane from the backside of the ribs. This can be done by cutting just through the membrane in an X pattern and working a paper towel between the membrane and the ribs to pull it off.

3. Coat the ribs on both sides with mustard and season them with the rub. Using your hands, work the rub into the meat.

4. Place the ribs directly on the grill grate and smoke until their internal temperature reaches between 190°F and 200°F.

5. Remove the racks from the grill and cut into individual ribs. Serve immediately.

82.   Kalbi Beef Ribs

Servings: 6
Cooking Time: 23 Minutes
Ingredients:
- Thinly sliced beef ribs - 2 ½ lbs
- Soy sauce - ½ cup
- Brown sugar - ½ cup
- Rice wine or mirin - ⅛ cup
- Minced garlic - 2 tbsp
- Sesame oil - 1 tbsp
- Grated onion - ⅛ cup

Directions:
1.   In a medium-sized bowl, mix the mirin, soy sauce, sesame oil, brown sugar, garlic, and grated onion.
2.   Add the ribs to the bowl to marinate and cover it properly with cling wrap. Put it in the refrigerator for up to 6 hours.
3.   Once you remove the marinated ribs from the refrigerator, immediately put them on the grill. Close the grill quickly, so no heat is lost. Also, make sure the grill is preheated well before you place the ribs on it.
4.   Cook on one side for 4 minutes and then flip it. Cook the other side for 4 minutes.
5.   Pull it out once it looks fully cooked. Serve it with rice or any other side dish
Nutrition Info: Carbohydrates: 22 g Protein: 28 g Fat: 6 g Sodium: 1213 mg Cholesterol: 81 mg

83.   Smoked Lamb Shoulder

Servings: 6

Cooking Time: 4 Hours

Ingredients:

- 8 pounds lamb shoulder, fat trimmed
- 2 tablespoons olive oil
- Salt as needed
- For the Rub:
- 1 tablespoon dried oregano
- 2 tablespoons salt
- 1 tablespoon crushed dried bay leaf
- 1 tablespoon sugar
- 2 tablespoons dried crushed sage
- 1 tablespoon dried thyme
- 1 tablespoon ground black pepper
- 1 tablespoon dried basil
- 1 tablespoon dried rosemary
- 1 tablespoon dried parsley

Directions:

1.   Switch on the grill, fill the grill hopper with cherry flavored wood pellets, power the grill on by using the control panel, select 'smoke' on the temperature dial, or set the temperature to 250 degrees F and let it preheat for a minimum of 5 minutes.

2.   Meanwhile, prepare the rub and for this, take a small bowl, place all of its ingredients in it and stir until mixed.

3.   Brush lamb with oil and then sprinkle with prepared rub until evenly coated.

4.   When the grill has preheated, open the lid, place lamb should on the grill grate fat-side up, shut the grill and smoke for 3 hours.

5.   Then change the smoking temperature to 325 degrees F and continue smoking to 1 hour until fat renders, and the internal temperature reaches 195 degrees F.

6.   When done, wrap lamb should in aluminum foil and let it rest for 20 minutes.

7.   Pull lamb shoulder by using two forks and then serve.

Nutrition Info: Calories: 300 Cal ;Fat: 24 g ;Carbs: 0 g ;Protein: 19 g ;Fiber: 0 g

84.   Wood Pellet Smoked Pulled Lamb Sliders

Servings: 7

Cooking Time: 7 Hours

Ingredients:

- For the Lamb's shoulder
- 5 lb lamb shoulder, boneless
- 1/2 cup olive oil
- 1/4 cup dry rub
- 10 oz spritz
- The Dry Rub
- 1/3 cup kosher salt
- 1/3 cup pepper, ground
- 1-1/3 cup garlic, granulated
- The Spritz
- 4 oz Worcestershire sauce
- 6 oz apple cider vinegar

Directions:

1.   Preheat the wood pellet smoker with a water bath to 250 F.
2.   Trim any fat from the lamb then rub with oil and dry rub.
3.   Place the lamb on the smoker for 90 minutes then spritz with a spray bottle every 30 minutes until the internal temperature reaches 165 F.
4.   Transfer the lamb shoulder to a foil pan with the remaining spritz liquid and cover tightly with foil.
5.   Place back in the smoker and smoke until the internal temperature reaches 200 F.
6.   Remove from the smoker and let rest for 30 minutes before pulling the lamb and serving with slaw, bun, or aioli. Enjoy

Nutrition Info: Calories 339, Total Fat 22, Saturated fat 7g, Total Carbs 16g, Net Carbs 15g, Protein 18g, Sugar 2g, Fiber 1g, Sodium: 459mg

85.   Strip Steak With Onion Sauce

Servings: 4
Cooking Time: 1 Hour
Ingredients:
- 2 New York strip steaks
- Prime rib rub
- ½ lb. bacon, chopped
- 1 onion, sliced
- 1/4 cup brown sugar
- 1/2 tablespoon balsamic vinegar
- 3 tablespoons brewed coffee
- 1/4 cup apple juice

Directions:
1. Sprinkle both sides of steaks with prime rib rub.
2. Set the wood pellet grill to 350 degrees F.
3. Preheat for 15 minutes while the lid is closed.
4. Place a pan over the grill.
5. Cook the bacon until crispy.
6. Transfer to a plate.
7. Cook the onion in the bacon drippings for 10 minutes.
8. Stir in brown sugar and cook for 20 minutes.
9. Add the rest of the ingredients and cook for 20 minutes.
10. Grill the steaks for 5 minutes per side.
11. Serve with the onion and bacon mixture.
12. Tips: Ensure steak is in room temperature before seasoning.

86.   Grilled Lamb Burgers

Servings: 5

Cooking Time: 15 Minutes

Ingredients:

- 1 1/4 pounds of ground lamb.
- 1 egg.
- 1 teaspoon of dried oregano.
- 1 teaspoon of dry sherry.
- 1 teaspoon of white wine vinegar.
- 4 minced cloves of garlic.
- Red pepper
- 1/2 cup of chopped green onions.
- 1 tablespoon of chopped mint.
- 2 tablespoons of chopped cilantro.
- 2 tablespoons of dry bread crumbs.
- 1/8 teaspoon of salt to taste.
- 1/4 teaspoon of ground black pepper to taste.
- 5 hamburger buns.

Directions:

1.   Preheat a Wood Pellet Smoker or Grill to 350-450 degrees F then grease it grates. Using a large mixing bowl, add in all the ingredients on the list aside from the buns then mix properly to combine with clean hands. Make about five patties out of the mixture then set aside.

2.   Place the lamb patties on the preheated grill and cook for about seven to nine minutes turning only once until an inserted thermometer reads 160 degrees F. Serve the lamb burgers on the hamburger, add your favorite toppings and enjoy.

Nutrition Info: Calories: 376 Cal Fat: 18.5 g Carbohydrates: 25.4 g Protein: 25.5 g Fiber: 1.6 g

87.   The Perfect T-bones

Servings: 4

Cooking Time: 30 Minutes

Ingredients:

- 4 (1½- to 2-inch-thick) T-bone steaks
- 2 tablespoons olive oil
- 1 batch Espresso Brisket Rub or Chili-Coffee Rub

Directions:

1.   Supply your with wood pellets and follow the start-up procedure. Preheat the grill, with the lid closed, to 500°F.

2.   Coat the steaks all over with olive oil and season both sides with the rub. Using your hands, work the rub into the meat.

3.   Place the steaks directly on a grill grate and smoke until their internal temperature reaches 135°F for rare, 145°F for medium-rare, and 155°F for well-done. Remove the steaks from the grill and serve hot.

88. Glorious Pork Back Ribs

Servings: 16

Cooking Time: 5 Hours

Ingredients:

- ¼ C. yellow honey mustard
- ¼ C. brown sugar
- 1/3 C. paprika
- ¼ C. garlic powder
- ¼ C. onion powder
- 2 tbsp. chipotle chili pepper flakes
- 1 tbsp. ground cumin
- Salt and freshly ground black pepper, to taste
- 2 tbsp. dried parsley flakes
- 8 lb. pork baby back ribs, silver skin removed

Directions:

1. In a bowl, add all ingredients except for ribs and mix well.
2. Rub the pork ribs with spice mixture generously.
3. Set the temperature of Grill to 200 degrees F and preheat with closed lid for 15 minutes, using charcoal.
4. Arrange the ribs onto the grill and cook for about 2 hours.
5. Remove the ribs from grill and wrap in heavy duty foil.
6. Cook for about 2 hours.
7. Remove the foil and cook for about 1 hour more.
8. Remove the ribs from grill and place onto a cutting board for about 10-15 minutes before serving.

Nutrition Info: Calories per serving: 659; Carbohydrates: 7.8g; Protein: 61.1g; Fat: 40.7g; Sugar: 4.4g; Sodium: 186mg; Fiber: 1.5g

89.   Wood Pellet Grilled Tenderloin With Fresh Herb Sauce

Servings: 4
Cooking Time: 15 Minutes
Ingredients:
- Pork
- 1 pork tenderloin, silver skin removed and dried
- BBQ seasoning
- Fresh herb sauce
- 1 handful basil, fresh
- 1/4 tbsp garlic powder
- 1/3 cup olive oil
- 1/2 tbsp kosher salt

Directions:
1.   Preheat the wood pellet grill to medium heat.
2.   Coat the pork with BBQ seasoning then cook on semi-direct heat of the grill. Turn the pork regularly to ensure even cooking.
3.   Cook until the internal temperature is 145°F. Remove from the grill and let it rest for 10 minutes.
4.   Meanwhile, make the herb sauce by pulsing all the sauce ingredients in a food processor. Pulse for a few times or until well chopped.
5.   Slice the pork diagonally and spoon the sauce on top. Serve and enjoy.

Nutrition Info: Calories 300, Total fat 22g, Saturated fat 4g, Total Carbs 13g, Net Carbs 12g, Protein 14g, Sugar 10g, Fiber 1g, Sodium: 791mg

90.   Togarashi Pork Tenderloin

Servings: 4

Cooking Time: 25 Minutes

Ingredients:

- 1 pork tenderloin
- 1/2 tbsp. kosher salt
- 1/4 cup Togarashi seasoning

Directions:

1. Trim off any silver skin on the pork tenderloin then sprinkle salt and togarashi seasoning evenly.
2. Preheat the to 400F.
3. Cook the pork for 25 minutes or until the internal temperature reaches 145F.
4. Remove the pork from the and let rest for 10 minutes before slicing and serving.

Nutrition Info: Calories 390, Total fat 19g, Saturated fat 4g, Total carbs 14g, Net carbs 11g Protein 40g, Sugars 8g, Fiber 3g, Sodium 420mg

91.   Greek-style Roast Leg Of Lamb

Servings: 12
Cooking Time: 1 Hour And 30 Minutes
Ingredients:

- 7 pounds leg of lamb, bone-in, fat trimmed
- 2 lemons, juiced
- 8 cloves of garlic, peeled, minced
- Salt as needed
- Ground black pepper as needed
- 1 teaspoon dried oregano
- 1 teaspoon dried rosemary
- 6 tablespoons olive oil

Directions:

1.   Make a small cut into the meat of lamb by using a paring knife, then stir together garlic, oregano, and rosemary and stuff this paste into the slits of the lamb meat.

2.   Take a roasting pan, place lamb in it, then rub with lemon juice and olive oil, cover with a plastic wrap and let marinate for a minimum of 8 hours in the refrigerator.

3.   When ready to cook, switch on the grill, fill the grill hopper with oak flavored wood pellets, power the grill on by using the control panel, select 'smoke' on the temperature dial, or set the temperature to 400 degrees F and let it preheat for a minimum of 15 minutes.

4.   Meanwhile, remove the lamb from the refrigerator, bring it to room temperature, uncover it and then season well with salt and black pepper.

5.   When the grill has preheated, open the lid, place food on the grill grate, shut the grill, and smoke for 30 minutes.

6.   Change the smoking temperature to 350 degrees F and then continue smoking for 1 hour until the internal temperature reaches 140 degrees F.

7.   When done, transfer lamb to a cutting board, let it rest for 15 minutes, then cut it into slices and serve.

Nutrition Info: Calories: 168 Cal ;Fat: 10 g ;Carbs: 2 g ;Protein: 17 g ;Fiber: 0.7 g

92. 2-ingredients Filet Mignon

Servings: 2

Cooking Time: 10 Minutes

Ingredients:

- 2 filet mignons
- Salt and freshly ground black pepper, to taste

Directions:

1. Set the temperature of Grill to 450 degrees F and preheat with closed lid for 15 minutes.
2. Season the steaks with salt and black pepper generously.
3. Place the filet mignons onto the grill and grill and cook for about 5 minutes per side.
4. Remove from grill and serve immediately.

Nutrition Info: Calories per serving: 254; Carbohydrates: 0g; Protein: 39.8g; Fat: 9.3g; Sugar: 0g; Sodium: 161mg; Fiber: 0g

Servings: 5

Cooking Time: 8 Hours

Ingredients:

- 3 lbs beef short ribs
- 2 tbsp sugar
- 3/4 cup water
- 1 tbsp ground black pepper
- 3 tbsp white vinegar
- 2 tbsp sesame oil
- 3 tbsp soy sauce
- 6 cloves garlic, minced
- 1/3 cup light brown sugar
- 1/2 yellow onion, finely chopped

Directions:

1. Combine soy sauce, water, and vinegar in a bowl. Mix and whisk in brown sugar, white sugar, pepper, sesame oil, garlic, and onion. Whisk until the sugars have completely dissolved

2. Pour marinade into large bowl or baking pan with high sides. Dunk the short ribs in the marinade, coating completely. Cover marinaded short ribs with plastic wrap and refrigerate for 6 to 12 hours3. Preheat pellet grill to 225°F.

3. Remove plastic wrap from ribs and pull ribs out of marinade. Shake off any excess marinade and dispose of the contents left in the bowl.

4. Place ribs on grill and cook for about 6-8 hours, until ribs reach an internal temperature of 203°F. Measure using a probe meat thermometer

5. Once ribs reach temperature, remove from grill and allow to rest for about 20 minutes. Slice, serve, and enjoy!

94.   Blackened Pork Chops

Servings: 6
Cooking Time: 20 Minutes
Ingredients:
- 6 pork chops
- 1/4 cup blackening seasoning
- Salt and pepper

Directions:
1. Preheat your to 375F.
2. Generously season the pork chops with the blackening seasoning, salt, and pepper.
3. Place the chops on the grill and cook for 8 minutes on one side then flip.
4. Cook until the internal temperature reaches 1420F.
5. Let the pork chops rest for 10 minutes before slicing and serving.

Nutrition Info: Calories 333, Total fat 18g, Saturated fat 6g, Total carbs 1g, Net carbs 0g Protein 40g, Sugars 0g, Fiber 1g, Sodium 3175mg

95.   Bbq Brisket

Servings: 8
Cooking Time: 10 Hours
Ingredients:
- 1 beef brisket, about 12 pounds
- Beef rub as needed

Directions:
1.   Season beef brisket with beef rub until well coated, place it in a large plastic bag, seal it and let it marinate for a minimum of 12 hours in the refrigerator.
2.   When ready to cook, switch on the grill, fill the grill hopper with hickory flavored wood pellets, power the grill on by using the control panel, select 'smoke' on the temperature dial, or set the temperature to 225 degrees F and let it preheat for a minimum of 15 minutes.
3.   When the grill has preheated, open the lid, place marinated brisket on the grill grate fat-side down, shut the grill, and smoke for 6 hours until the internal temperature reaches 160 degrees F.
4.   Then wrap the brisket in foil, return it back to the grill grate and cook for 4 hours until the internal temperature reaches 204 degrees F.
5.   When done, transfer brisket to a cutting board, let it rest for 30 minutes, then cut it into slices and serve.

Nutrition Info: Calories: 328 Cal ;Fat: 21 g ;Carbs: 0 g ;Protein: 32 g ;Fiber: - g

96.   Sweet And Hot Bbq Ribs

Servings: 4
Cooking Time: 5 Hours And 10 Minutes

Ingredients:

- 2 racks of pork ribs, bone-in, membrane removed
- 6 ounces pork and poultry rub
- 8 ounces apple juice
- 16 ounces sweet and heat BBQ sauce

Directions:

1.   Sprinkle pork and poultry rub on all sides of pork ribs until evenly coated, rub well and marinate for a minimum of 30 minutes.
2.   When ready to cook, switch on the grill, fill the grill hopper with pecan flavored wood pellets, power the grill on by using the control panel, select 'smoke' on the temperature dial, or set the temperature to 225 degrees F and let it preheat for a minimum of 15 minutes.
3.   When the grill has preheated, open the lid, place pork ribs on the grill grate bone-side down, shut the grill and smoke for 1 hour, spraying with 10 ounces of apple juice frequently.
4.   Then wrap ribs in aluminum foil, pour in remaining 6 ounces of apple juice, and wrap tightly.
5.   Return wrapped ribs onto the grill grate meat-side down, shut the grill and smoke for 3 to 4 hours until internal temperature reaches 203 degrees F.
6.   Remove wrapped ribs from the grill, uncover it and then brush well with the sauce.
7.   Return pork ribs onto the grill grate and then grill for 10 minutes until glazed.
8.   When done, transfer ribs to a cutting board, let rest for 10 minutes, then cut it into slices and serve.

Nutrition Info: Calories: 250.8 Cal ;Fat: 16.3 g ;Carbs: 6.5 g ;Protein: 18.2 g ;Fiber: 0.2 g

97.   Wine Braised Lamb Shank

Servings: 2
Cooking Time: 10 Hours
Ingredients:
- 2 (1¼-lb.) lamb shanks
- 1-2 C. water
- ¼ C. brown sugar
- 1/3 C. rice wine
- 1/3 C. soy sauce
- 1 tbsp. dark sesame oil
- 4 (1½x½-inch) orange zest strips
- 2 (3-inch long) cinnamon sticks
- 1½ tsp. Chinese five-spice powder

Directions:
1.   Set the temperature of Grill to 225-250 degrees F and preheat with closed lid for 15 minutes. , using charcoal and soaked apple wood chips.
2.   With a sharp knife, pierce each lamb shank at many places.
3.   In a bowl, add remaining all ingredients and mix until sugar is dissolved.
4.   In a large foil pan, place the lamb shanks and top with sugar mixture evenly.
5.   Place the foil pan onto the grill and cook for about 8-10 hours, flipping after every 30 minutes. (If required, add enough water to keep the liquid ½-inch over).
6.   Remove from the grill and serve hot.

Nutrition Info: Calories per serving: 1200; Carbohydrates: 39.7g; Protein: 161.9g; Fat: 48.4; Sugar: 29g; Sodium: 2000mg; Fiber: 0.3g

98.   Competition Style Bbq Pork Ribs

Servings: 6

Cooking Time: 2 Hours

Ingredients:

- 2 racks of St. Louis-style ribs
- 1 cup Pork and Poultry Rub
- 1/8 cup brown sugar
- 4 tablespoons butter
- 4 tablespoons agave
- 1 bottle Sweet and Heat BBQ Sauce

Directions:

1.   Place the ribs in working surface and remove the thin film of connective tissues covering it. In a smaller bowl, combine the Pork and Poultry Rub, brown sugar, butter, and agave. Mix until well combined.

2.   Massage the rub onto the ribs and allow to rest in the fridge for at least 2 hours.

3.   When ready to cook, fire the Grill to 225F. Use desired wood pellets when cooking the ribs. Close the lid and preheat for 15 minutes.

4.   Place the ribs on the grill grate and close the lid. Smoke for 1 hour and 30 minutes. Make sure to flip the ribs halfway through the cooking time.

5.   Ten minutes before the cooking time ends, brush the ribs with BBQ sauce.

6.   Remove from the grill and allow to rest before slicing.

Nutrition Info: Calories per serving: 399 ; Protein: 47.2g; Carbs: 3.5g; Fat: 20.5g Sugar: 2.3g

99.   Cheesy Lamb Burgers

Servings: 4
Cooking Time: 20 Minutes
Ingredients:
- 2 lb. ground lamb
- 1 C. Parmigiano-Reggiano cheese, grated
- Salt and freshly ground black pepper, to taste

Directions:
1. Set the temperature of Grill to 425 degrees F and preheat with closed lid for 15 minutes.
2. In a bowl, add all ingredients and mix well.
3. Make 4 (¾-inch thick) patties from mixture.
4. With your thumbs, make a shallow but wide depression in each patty.
5. Arrange the patties onto the grill, depression-side down and cook for about 8 minutes.
6. Flip and cook for about 8-10 minutes.
7. Serve immediately.

Nutrition Info: Calories per serving: 502; Carbohydrates: 0g; Protein: 71.7g; Fat: 22.6g; Sugar: 0g; Sodium: 331mg; Fiber: 0g

100. Deliciously Spicy Rack Of Lamb

Servings: 6
Cooking Time: 3 Hours
Ingredients:
- 2 tbsp. paprika
- ½ tbsp. coriander seeds
- 1 tsp. cumin seeds
- 1 tsp. ground allspice
- 1 tsp. lemon peel powder
- Salt and freshly ground black pepper, to taste
- 2 (1½-lb.) rack of lamb ribs, trimmed

Directions:
1. Set the temperature of Grill to 225 degrees F and preheat with closed lid for 15 minutes.
2. In a coffee grinder, add all ingredients except rib racks and grind into a powder.
3. Coat the rib racks with spice mixture generously.
4. Arrange the rib racks onto the grill and cook for about 3 hours.
5. Remove the rib racks from grill and place onto a cutting board for about 10-15 minutes before slicing.
6. With a sharp knife, cut the rib racks into equal-sized individual ribs and serve.

Nutrition Info: Calories per serving: 545; Carbohydrates: 1.7g; Protein: 64.4g; Fat: 29.7g; Sugar: 0.3g; Sodium: 221mg; Fiber: 1g

CPSIA information can be obtained
at www.ICGtesting.com
Printed in the USA
LVHW101216270121
677614LV00019B/1076